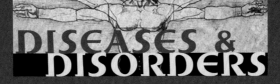

DISEASES & DISORDERS

Speech Disorders

Wendy Lanier

LUCENT BOOKS
A part of Gale, Cengage Learning

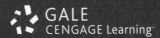

Detroit • New York • San Francisco • New Haven, Conn • Waterville, Maine • London

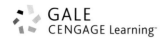
GALE
CENGAGE Learning™

© 2010 Gale, Cengage Learning

LIBRARY OF CONGRESS CATALOGING-IN-PUBLICATION DATA

Lanier, Wendy, 1963-
  Speech disorders / by Wendy Lanier.
    p. cm. -- (Diseases & disorders)
  Includes bibliographical references and index.
  ISBN 978-1-4205-0221-3 (hardcover)
  1. Speech disorders--Popular works. I. Title.
  RC423.L3395 2010
  616.85'5--dc22

                                                    2009040807

Lucent Books
27500 Drake Rd.
Farmington Hills, MI 48331

ISBN-13: 978-1-4205-0221-3
ISBN-10: 1-4205-0221-2

Printed in the United States of America
2 3 4 5 6 7 14 13 12 11 10

Printed by Bang Printing, Brainerd, MN, 2nd Ptg., 01/2011

Table of Contents

"The Most Difficult Puzzles Ever Devised"

Charles Best, one of the pioneers in the search for a cure for diabetes, once explained what it is about medical research that intrigued him so. "It's not just the gratification of knowing one is helping people," he confided, "although that probably is a more heroic and selfless motivation. Those feelings may enter in, but truly, what I find best is the feeling of going toe to toe with nature, of trying to solve the most difficult puzzles ever devised. The answers are there somewhere, those keys that will solve the puzzle and make the patient well. But how will those keys be found?"

Since the dawn of civilization, nothing has so puzzled people—and often frightened them, as well—as the onset of illness in a body or mind that had seemed healthy before. A seizure, the inability of a heart to pump, the sudden deterioration of muscle tone in a small child—being unable to reverse such conditions or even to understand why they occur was unspeakably frustrating to healers. Even before there were names for such conditions, even before they were understood at all, each was a reminder of how complex the human body was, and how vulnerable.

While our grappling with understanding diseases has been frustrating at times, it has also provided some of humankind's most heroic accomplishments. Alexander Fleming's accidental discovery in 1928 of a mold that could be turned into penicillin has resulted in the saving of untold millions of lives. The isolation of the enzyme insulin has reversed what was once a death sentence for anyone with diabetes. There have been great strides in combating conditions for which there is not yet a cure, too. Medicines can help AIDS patients live longer, diagnostic tools such as mammography and ultrasounds can help doctors find tumors while they are treatable, and laser surgery techniques have made the most intricate, minute operations routine.

This "toe-to-toe" competition with diseases and disorders is even more remarkable when seen in a historical continuum. An astonishing amount of progress has been made in a very short time. Just two hundred years ago, the existence of germs as a cause of some diseases was unknown. In fact, it was less than 150 years ago that a British surgeon named Joseph Lister had difficulty persuading his fellow doctors that washing their hands before delivering a baby might increase the chances of a healthy delivery (especially if they had just attended to a diseased patient)!

Each book in Lucent's Diseases and Disorders series explores a disease or disorder and the knowledge that has been accumulated (or discarded) by doctors through the years. Each book also examines the tools used for pinpointing a diagnosis, as well as the various means that are used to treat or cure a disease. Finally, new ideas are presented—techniques or medicines that may be on the horizon.

Frustration and disappointment are still part of medicine, for not every disease or condition can be cured or prevented. But the limitations of knowledge are being pushed outward constantly; the "most difficult puzzles ever devised" are finding challengers every day.

When Communicating Is a Problem

In a crowded mall or in the hallways at school, sounds of conversation fill the air. The most common way humans communicate is by talking. For most people the act of vocalizing their thoughts is effortless. They think of what they want to say and then say it. But for nearly 17 percent of the U.S. population, the ability to put thoughts into words is impaired by some type of communication disorder.

Current statistics indicate that 1.3 million children in the United States have a noticeable speech problem before first grade. Add to that the number of speech difficulties that are the result of accidents or illness and the number increases to about 8 million Americans with some form of language impairment. These impairments range from mild (hardly noticeable) to severe (crippling a person's ability to communicate).

Humans communicate through verbal sounds that have specific meanings. While normal speech appears effortless, it is actually produced by carefully choreographed movements of the head, neck, chest, and abdomen. An injury or defect at any one of these sites can affect normal speech.

Speech disorders are many and varied. Most children, for example, go through phases of mispronouncing specific sounds. Their speech errors are considered a problem when they continue past a certain age. A person with a hearing loss or who is deaf typically has difficulty acquiring speech and usually exhibits speech disorders related to the inability to hear. Sometimes injuries or illnesses such as stroke or Alzheimer's disease can cause a person who has always had normal speech to develop difficulties. The type of disorder and the age of onset usually determine whether a return to normal speech is possible.

Individuals who suffer from speech disorders are often treated as mentally inferior even though they may have an IQ well above normal. They may find themselves the subjects of jokes, objects of curious stares, ridiculed in public, or victims of impatient listeners who refuse to wait for them to finish speaking.

Fortunately, most speech disorders can be treated. Professionals known as speech pathologists and special therapists are trained to identify types of speech problems and design therapy methods to help reduce or eliminate their effects. Individuals who work in this field can be found in a variety of

A young boy with a speech disorder works with a speech therapist to help him pronounce words. Speech disorders among children are many and varied.

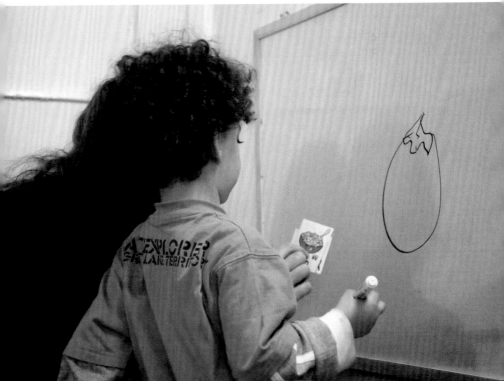

settings. They work in hospitals, schools, clinics, and other settings with children and adults who are experiencing difficulty communicating clearly.

Although not life threatening, speech disorders are usually difficult to live with. People with speech disorders must work hard to improve their speech or find an alternative means of communication while still maintaining a positive outlook on life. Those who refuse to allow their disorder to keep them from interacting with others develop a kind of perseverance and can-do attitude that serves them well in every area of their lives.

CHAPTER ONE

What Is a Speech Disorder?

Speech disorders affect the way a person talks. A person with a speech disorder usually knows exactly what they want to say and what is appropriate for the situation, but they have trouble producing the sounds to communicate it effectively.

Speech disorders include a variety of conditions that affect children and adults alike. They can range from trouble pronouncing a specific letter or sound to the inability to produce any understandable speech. Some are the result of a physical deformity. Others are the result of damage to the speech mechanism (larynx, lips, teeth, tongue, and palate) caused by injury or diseases, such as cancer. Often, however, the cause of a speech disorder is not known.

Speech Language Pathology

Speech language pathology is the study of the disorders that affect speech, language, cognition, voice, swallowing, and the corrective treatment of the physical or cognitive issues that may be causing them. Speech language pathologists, sometimes called speech therapists or SLPs, work with patients to achieve or restore normal speech if possible.

In general, SLPs work with three basic types of speech disorders: fluency disorders, articulation disorders, and voice disorders.

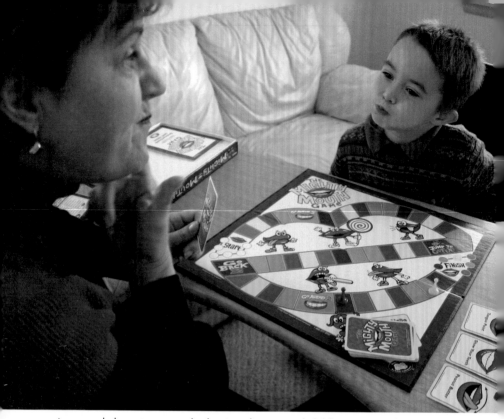

A speech language pathologist shows a child how to make speech sounds to improve his pronunciation during a therapy session.

Fluency Disorders

Fluency disorders are related to the smoothness or rhythm of speech. A person with a fluency disorder may hesitate, repeat words, or prolong certain sounds, syllables, words, or phrases. Stuttering and cluttering are types of fluency disorders.

A well-known example of someone who exhibits a fluency disorder is Porky Pig. His "Th- th- th- th- that's all folks!" at the end of a Warner Brothers cartoon is a familiar part of American pop culture. The chubby little pig with the pronounced stutter is a beloved character—the star of hundreds of cartoons since he was first introduced in 1935. Although stuttering may be an endearing quality for Porky, those who suffer with this type of fluency disorder in the real world find it a tremendous challenge.

Fluency disorders are especially common among young children. In most cases, children progress through this disfluency phase in a few months. As they learn to compose complex

What Is the "Language" in Speech Language Pathology?

Most speech professionals who treat communication disorders refer to their work as speech/language therapy. While the two are usually treated together, language disorders are not quite the same thing as speech disorders. Language disorders have to do with a person's ability to understand, form, or use words correctly. This can occur in both verbal and nonverbal communication. The inability to find and use the right words or gestures at the appropriate time indicates a problem with the mental, not physical, process of language. Speech and language disorders often occur together, making it almost impossible at times to distinguish between the two.

Aphasia is a common language disorder that often appears after a stroke. This affects a person's ability to comprehend what they hear or compose what they want to say. While it does not have any effect on the person's physical capability to produce speech, he or she may spend long moments searching for the right word or have difficulty formulating a sentence that makes sense. In some cases a person may feel as though everyone else is speaking a foreign language and everything he or she reads is gibberish. Or, a person may understand what is said but is unable to produce anything but garbled speech in response.

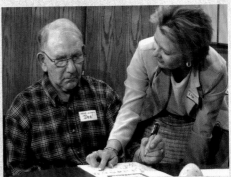

A speech language therapist works with a stroke patient who has aphasia to help him compose his thoughts before he speaks them aloud.

statements, questions, or commands, children often interject extra words or sounds between words (adding "uh" or "you know"), revise or change a sentence ("Mom went—Mom drove to the store"), repeat certain phrases ("we are going, we are going home"), or repeat a particular word ("I—I—I want that").

While childhood fluency errors are common, pediatricians still monitor them closely. A disfluency phase that lasts longer than a few months may require the help of an SLP. If no effort is made to correct it, the condition could continue and become even worse by adulthood.

Fluency disorders that persist past the preschool years are particularly vexing because they can influence how well a child adjusts to school and other social situations outside the home. Little is known about the cause of such disorders. Adults who struggle with fluency disorders often have difficulty with social interactions because they are embarrassed by their inability to speak smoothly. They may withdraw from social interaction as much as possible if people with whom they attempt to communicate are unkind or impatient with their efforts. Although fluency disorders are generally not considered a serious medical problem, they have the potential to greatly influence a person's education, vocation, and emotional well-being. One man notes, "For many years I had things to say and I refused to try. I refused to even consider making the choice to say them."[1]

Articulation Disorders

A second type of speech disorder involves the formation or articulation of words. Articulation is achieved through the use of the lips, tongue, teeth, and palate. In some cases an injury or congenital birth defect affects one or more of these body parts and leads to an inability to pronounce words correctly. For example, a small child who loses his or her front teeth all at once may develop a lisp. In this case the disorder is only temporary. But in the case of oral cancer patients who have had a part of their jaw removed, the challenges of articulating words are much more pronounced and more difficult to overcome.

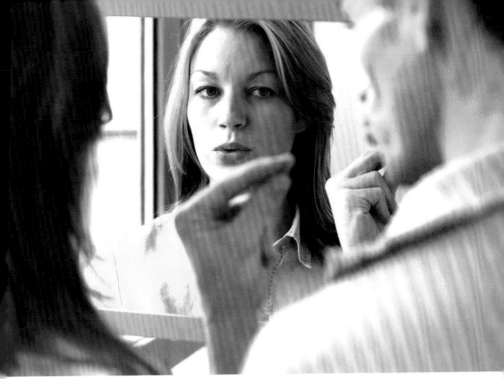

A woman is led through an articulation exercise by a speech pathologist to improve her speech.

A person with an articulation disorder typically has trouble pronouncing sounds or makes errors in the way these sounds are strung together. One sound might be substituted for another ("wabbit" for "rabbit"), omitted altogether ("and" for "hand"), or distorted by mispronouncing it ("ship" for "sip"). The most common error sounds include "s," "l," and "r."

Some articulation errors are the result of regional dialect or slang. Certain letter omissions or substitutions may be so common they are hardly noticed within a certain region or group. It is only when a person travels outside their region or begins interacting with people outside his or her usual group that his or her articulation becomes noticeable.

People in some parts of the United States, for example, tend to omit the letter "r" in phrases such as "pahk the cah" for "park the car." In other regions it is common to leave off the final "g" in a word ending in "ing" such as "goin" for "going" or "tellin" for "telling." A regional or ethnic dialect is not considered a disorder unless it is perceived to be by the speaker.

SLPs often work with individuals who wish to reduce the effects of an accent, but only at the speaker's request.

The effects of an articulation disorder do not usually keep a speaker from being understood; however, they can impact the way a listener reacts. Whether listeners are aware of it or not, many make judgments about a speaker's intelligence based on speech patterns. An adult with a lisp, for example, may have difficulty getting listeners to take him or her seriously.

When children are small, articulation errors are common. In fact, they may seem cute, but allowing them to go unchecked establishes poor speech habits. SLP Nancy Lucker-Lazerson, believes early intervention is key. "Traditional thinking has been that some articulation errors are developmental in nature ([for example,] s, l, r) and that children may not be ready to address them in therapy until a specific age (typically 7 or 8). However, current research has disproved the idea of developmental norms for articulation."[2] She is a firm believer that the earlier therapy begins, the more successful it will be.

Although articulation errors may not keep children from being understood, errors that continue into school age can make the child a target for teasing and bullying. Sharon, mother of preschool-age Jordan, did not want her daughter to have that problem. She realized her daughter would need help in correcting her articulation errors since "Jordan used 'back' sounds for 'front' ones. She would say 'gog' instead of dog and 'Garah' for her sister Sarah."[3] As a result, Jordan was placed in speech therapy to help with articulation.

Usually, articulation errors are the easiest to remedy. Sometimes it is as simple as the speaker becoming aware of the error and making the corrections on his or her own. When this fails, speech therapy is an option.

Voice Disorders

A third type of speech disorder involves vocal pitch, quality (resonance), and/or loudness. A person with a voice disorder has a problem producing the sounds of speech. In some cases voice pitch may be monotonous or too high or too low for a person's age or gender. Sometimes listeners are startled by the harshness, hoarseness, or nasal quality of a person's voice. And occasionally the sheer loudness or resonance of a person's voice will cause heads to turn when he or she speaks.

Voice disorders are caused by damage, disease, or deformity of the larynx, or voice box. The larynx, a 2-inch (5cm) long, tube-shaped organ in the neck, creates the vibrations necessary to produce the sounds of speech. The outer wall of the larynx is a ring of cartilage. The muscles of the larynx are the vocal folds, two bands of leathery tissue inside the ring. In a relaxed state the folds remain open, and air passes through the opening silently.

Sound is produced when air is pushed up through the closed or partially closed vocal folds, causing them to vibrate. Changing the pitch of a sound requires tightening or relaxing the folds. Tightening the folds causes them to vibrate faster and produces a higher pitch. Relaxing the folds allows for the

This photo gives a close-up view of the vocal cords. Voice disorders can occur when the voice box, or larynx, is damaged by disease or deformity.

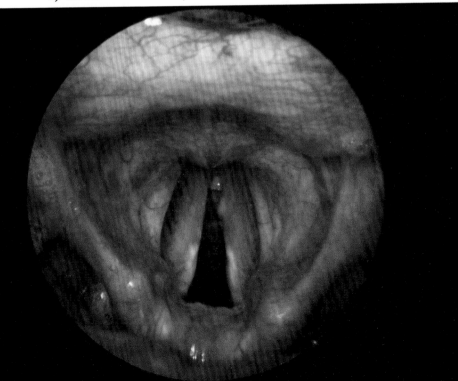

production of a lower pitch. An injury or illness can cause the vocal folds to vibrate improperly, resulting in a voice disorder. If the injury or illness is serious enough, such as in the case of advanced throat cancer, it may be necessary to remove the larynx altogether.

Voice disorders usually occur after a person has acquired speech. Colds, allergies, yelling for the home team, bronchitis, or exposure to an irritant such as household cleaners or paint can all lead to temporary voice disorders. The most common of these is mild laryngitis. However, conditions such as gastric reflux, cancer, and vocal abuse can lead to more serious and persistent voice disorders. The presence of tumors or cancer may require surgery to remove the entire larynx or some part of it.

The National Institute on Deafness and Other Communication Diseases estimates that approximately 7.5 million Americans suffer with some form of voice disorder. These disorders have the potential to negatively impact a person's social, emotional, and physical well-being. This is especially true of professionals who earn their living through speaking or singing. Although voice disorders associated with vocal abuse can be treated and reversed, other conditions have the potential to permanently damage a person's voice quality.

Speech Disorders in Children

In general, speech disorders are more common among children than adults. Children most often exhibit problems with articulation by mispronouncing words, lisping, or producing very nasal sounds as a result of a cleft lip or palate. Stuttering (a fluency disorder) and childhood apraxia of speech (a motor or movement disorder) are also common.

Sometimes children are born with conditions that make it difficult, if not impossible, to learn the complex process of speech. Deafness, cleft palate or lip, cerebral palsy, muscular dystrophy, Down's syndrome, and mental retardation affect how well, or even if, a child with any of these conditions can learn to speak. Although these cases are particularly disturbing,

What Are the "Normal" Stages of Learning to Speak?

Children who exhibit signs of a speech disorder may be able to make the necessary corrections on their own, but sometimes they require the help of speech therapy. Speech milestones include:

birth to 5 months: Infant reacts to sounds, turns toward source to watch, vocalizes pleasure and displeasure when spoken to.

6 to 11 months: Understands "no-no," babbles, communicates by actions or gestures, tries to repeat sounds.

12 to 17 months: Points, focuses on book or toy for two minutes, follows simple directions, answers simple questions nonverbally, clearly says two or three words as labels.

18 to 23 months: Enjoys being read to, follows simple commands, points to body parts, understands simple verbs (eat, sleep), pronounces most vowels and n, m, p, h, uses eight to ten words, makes animal sounds.

2 to 3 years: Uses at least forty words, knows spatial concepts (in, on) and pronouns (you, me, her), uses two- or three-word phrases and inflection, may not be understood by strangers.

3 to 4 years: Groups objects, identifies color, uses most speech sounds, describes use of objects, expresses feelings and ideas.

4 to 5 years: Understandable speech with mistakes, says two hundred to three hundred different words, uses some irregular verbs (ran, fell), tells how to do things, answers "why" questions.

5 years: Understands more than two thousand words, understands time sequence, carries out series of three directions, understands rhyming, uses eight or more words per sentence.

their incidence is quite low among the total population. Other conditions affecting speech development include poor rearing conditions, ear infections, child abuse, exposure to environmental toxins, illegal drug use by a parent, or the excessive use of alcohol, caffeine, or nicotine by a parent.

Without these risk factors, most childhood speech disorders disappear with age. Even if the disorder requires therapy, children often outgrow or overcome the disorder while they are still young. In most of these situations, the cause of the specific disorder is never known.

Speech Disorder in Adults

By contrast, speech disorders in adults are frequently acquired postlingually, meaning after speech has developed. The cause may be readily identified, but the effect can be far more devastating. Strokes, cancer, injury, or degenerative diseases can rob an adult of the ability to participate in a simple conversation. While therapy methods can help with adult speech disorders, a complete return to normal speech is rarely possible.

A veteran recovering from wounds practices breathing exercises with a speech pathologist to help alleviate the stress that causes stuttering.

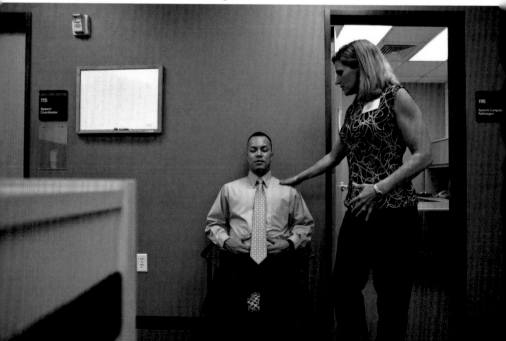

Common speech disorders in adults include fluency disorders like stuttering, voice disorders, and motor speech disorders, such as apraxia and dysarthria. Apraxia and dysarthria generally cause problems with articulation but can also contribute to voice or fluency issues.

Speech disorders include a wide range of issues. Some are more common than others. Some occur for no known reason while others are linked to specific genetic defects or diseases. No matter what the cause, a speech disorder has the potential to seriously affect a person's quality of life.

CHAPTER TWO

Common Speech Disorders

Although speech disorders can occur at any age, children are more likely to exhibit speech disorders than adults. The most severe are tied to congenital disorders that impair the natural development of speech. Others are relatively mild and usually disappear over time. Some speech disorders appear early in life and carry over into the adult years.

Stuttering

Perhaps the most common and easily recognized speech disorder is a fluency disorder called stuttering. Current statistics show that more than 3 million Americans and more than 15 million people worldwide are known to stutter. In the United States about 5 percent of adults report stuttering at some time in their life. Most of them began stuttering between the ages of two and six. In about 65 to 75 percent of the cases the stuttering stopped within two years of its onset; in 10 percent it disappeared within a few years after that. Only in about 1 percent of the cases did the stuttering continue into adulthood.

A person who stutters involuntarily repeats sounds and syllables. For example, a person may say "b-b-b-ball" for "ball," repeating the first letter several times before finishing the word. He or she may linger on one sound longer than is necessary, producing a voiced sound almost like a musical note. Or, they may interrupt the word they want to say with an involuntary pause by saying something like, "b' all."

People who stutter are usually self-conscious about their speech. They know very well that the sounds they are producing are not part of standard speech, but they are unable to control the flow. Those who stutter will often blink or contort their faces from the tension caused by their disorder. These involuntary movements only serve to increase the speaker's discomfort and may lead to more frequent stuttering.

Children who stutter will get so tense from the effort of speaking that they will often blink or contort their faces.

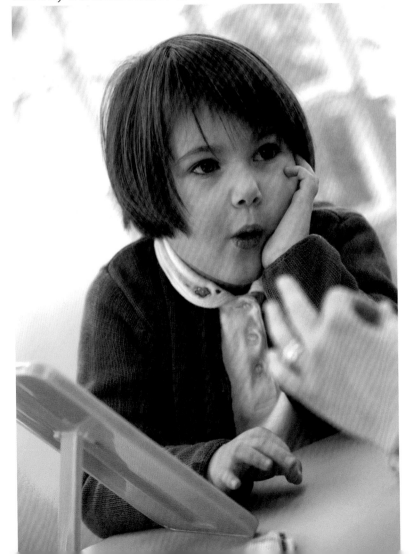

Pamela Mertz, a New York woman who has struggled with stuttering most of her life, describes her disorder as an embarrassment that, until recently, led her to stay quiet as much as possible. "The words were often there," she relates in an article for the International Stuttering Awareness Day Online Conference in 2008, "for I always knew what I wanted to say. Sometimes, I just couldn't get them out—like having a hand around my throat, squeezing the words in. When I tried to push, my speech became worse. No sound would come out, and I would be caught in an embarrassing block, which was even worse than stuttering."[4]

A Social Nightmare

Most people who stutter find they share the same nightmares. Situations that require them to speak publicly, on the phone, or to someone they do not know are all likely to dramatically increase their stress levels and, as a result, the frequency of their stuttering. Most people with a stuttering disorder quickly learn to avoid these situations as much as possible—a practice that can have negative results.

Walter H. Manning, a professor of audiology and speech language pathology at the University of Memphis and a stutterer himself, observes, "Because of my avoidance and caution with all things associated with speaking, stuttering prevented me from understanding who I was or knowing what I was capable of becoming. Decades later I began to understand that my lack of spontaneity in speaking also limited my spontaneity in thinking."[5]

Cause of Stuttering

Because stuttering can have such a profound impact on a person, much research has been done to determine the cause. Although the exact cause is still not known, researchers may be closing in on a possible answer. At this point, researchers know that boys are three to four times more likely to stutter than girls, but they do not know exactly why. They have also discovered that more than 50 percent of the people who stutter have a relative who stuttered at some point in his or her life. This suggests that stuttering may be genetic, possibly linked to a single gene.

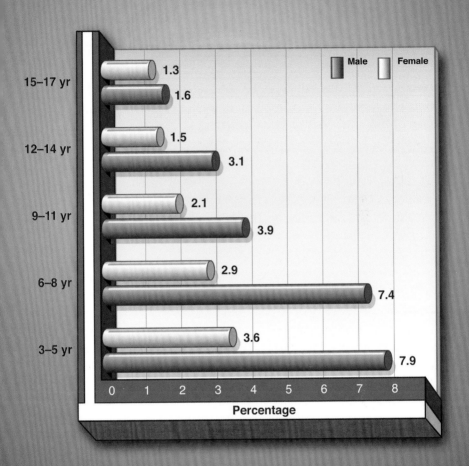

Frequency of Speech Disorders for Children Aged 3 to 17 (in a 12-month span)

Male / Female

Age	Male	Female
15–17 yr	1.3	1.6
12–14 yr	1.5	3.1
9–11 yr	2.1	3.9
6–8 yr	2.9	7.4
3–5 yr	3.6	7.9

Percentage

Taken from: National Institute on Deafness and Other Communication Disorders. Available online at www.nidcd.nih.gov/health/statistics/vsl/problems.htm.

What speech professionals do know at this point is that the treatment of stuttering is most effective when initiated in early childhood, although treatment at any age can help reduce the incidence. Meanwhile the research and treatment continues. Professor of speech language pathology Robert E. Owens Jr. and his coauthors of *Introduction to Communication Disorders: A*

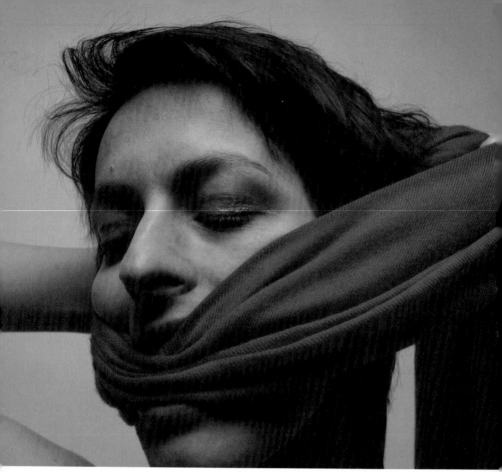

Stutterers have the same nightmares of not being able to speak publicly, on the phone, or to someone they do not know.

Lifespan Perspective believe that "solving the riddle of stuttering will undoubtedly require expertise from many specialists including SLPs, neurolinguists, geneticists, and medical specialists."[6]

Lisps

A lisp is an articulation disorder in which a person mispronounces the letters "s" and "z." A person may say "yeth" for "yes" or "that" for "sat." Sometimes a lisp is barely noticeable. In extreme cases, a person's tongue may actually protrude from the mouth during the formation of certain letters, producing a soft "th" sound. Although a lisp due to lost teeth is only temporary, one that carries over into school and adult years can be a source of embarrassment and teasing. Fortunately, lisps can usually be corrected.

Country Music Star Mel Tillis

Country Music Hall of Famer Mel Tillis began his career as a singer/songwriter in the early 1950s. Since that time he has earned honors as a Country Music Association (CMA) Entertainer of the Year, a two-time Broadcast Music, Inc. (BMI) Songwriter of the Decade winner, and has won a host of other awards. And he did it all in spite of his stuttering.

While in high school Mel realized he could sing without stuttering—a discovery that led him to choose a career in music. After a stint in the U.S. Air Force (where he experienced discrimination because of his stutter), Mel headed to Nashville to begin a career as a singer/songwriter.

At first Nashville music executives scoffed at the idea of a stuttering country singer, but soon his songwriting skills earned him a permanent job. When he first began singing he tried to avoid talking altogether. He was afraid people would laugh. When he expressed his fears to comedienne Minnie Pearl, she told him, "Let'em laugh. Goodness gracious, laughs are hard to get and I'm sure that they're laughing with you and not against you."

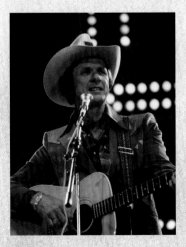

Following Minnie's lead, Mel began playing up his stuttering for laughs and telling stories about himself. He went on to become a popular singer, songwriter, and comedian.

Mel Tillis was perhaps the best-known stutterer in the 1970s and 1980s.

Causes of Lisps

Lisping can happen for a variety of reasons. Defects in the teeth or structure of the mouth, cleft palate, hearing loss, or an unconscious imitation of other lispers may contribute to the presence of a lisp. A person may even be unaware of a lisp until someone else points it out.

News interviewer Barbara Walters is one of many people with a lisp who have been successful in the communications business.

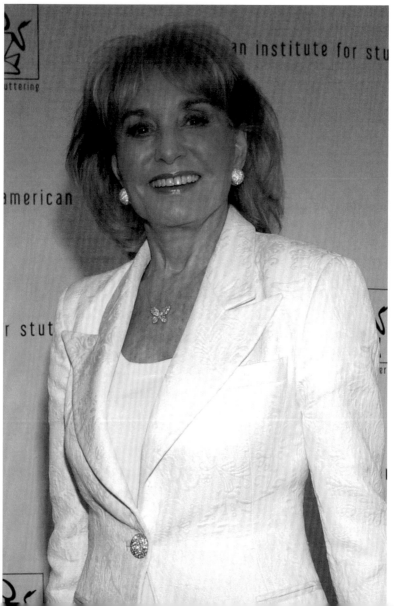

In a 2006 Internet video post, then twenty-five-year-old Tina expressed her shock and dismay at learning she had a lisp. This was "something that took me 25 years to find out—that nobody thought it was important enough to tell me," she says, "my family, my friends, my husband. Nobody. I had to record myself on video and then find out by watching the video. . . . You'd think that I'd be able to hear it, but I really didn't hear anything."[7]

In the absence of a physical cause, many people with lisps can often correct the problem on their own, but it usually takes months of retraining. Careful thought must be given to each sentence before it is spoken. When this does not work, speech therapy is another option.

Although lisping is a speech error, many adults choose to live with it. Successful adults with mild to moderate lisps can be found working in the field of communications and many other high-profile professions. Over the years, American pop culture has embraced characters and personalities such as Warner Brothers' Sylvester the cartoon cat, Cindy Brady of the 1970s-era sitcom *The Brady Bunch*, and news interviewer Barbara Walters—all with lisps.

In spite of this, some adults find lisping to be a source of embarrassment. Erika, a communication disorders major in college, shared her reason for wanting to work in her chosen field. "When I was a little girl, I can painfully remember being picked on by the other children about the way I spoke. My once cute lisp was no longer cute at 8. I was told that 'I talked like a baby' or sometimes the kids would mimic what I said in an exaggerated way." After moving to a new school where she received speech therapy, Erika was able to conquer her articulation problem. Today she wants to help others in similar situations. As she points out, "I know the hurt that accompanies the humiliation of being teased because you can't communicate properly."[8]

Dysarthria

Dysarthria is a group of neurologically related speech disorders. Known as motor speech disorders, dysarthrias are caused by lesions on the brain in areas responsible for planning, executing, and controlling the movements necessary for speech. This damage can cause speech muscles to become weak or paralyzed. Dysarthria is most common in people born with cerebral palsy (CP) or muscular dystrophy and adults who have experienced a stroke, tumor, or degenerative disease such as Parkinson's disease. People with dysarthria may experience speech issues ranging from only a slight hoarseness to an inability to speak at all.

Speech Affected by Dysarthria

Speech affected by dysarthria is slow, slurred, and difficult to understand due to errors in the articulation of consonants. Unlike some other speech disorders these errors are usually consistent and predictable. Other indications of dysarthria may include a voice that sounds as though the speaker is talking through his or her nose (due to the inability to control air flow), hoarseness, or a rapid rate of speech with a "mumbling" quality. However, the severity of the symptoms depends on the location and amount of damage to the nervous system. In extreme cases speech may not be possible, and the use of an alternative means of communication may be necessary.

Numbers of People Affected by Dysarthria

Because dysarthria is associated with so many health issues, it is difficult to determine how many people are actually affected by it. In addition, dysarthria can occur in conjunction with other types of speech disorders which affect the understanding of speech. Of the 6 to 8 million people in the United States who have some form of language impairment, as many as half may have some degree of dysarthria.

A Frustrating Disorder

The inability to control the movements necessary for speech is frustrating because it interferes with communication. Although difficult to understand, those who suffer with dysarthria are not necessarily mentally impaired. People who converse with

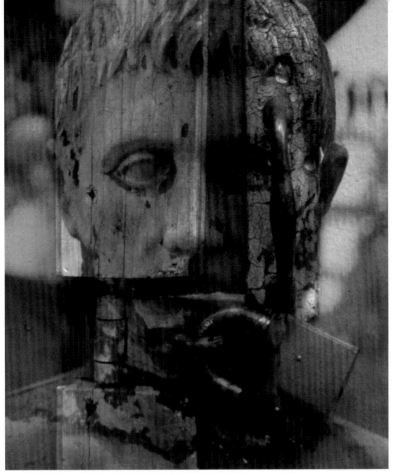

Dysarthria is a frustrating disorder because it interferes with a person's ability to communicate effectively.

them often assume the slurred speech and slow delivery are the result of diminished mental capacity, which is not true.

Kayla Smith, an adult with CP who works as an advocate for the disabled and blogs about the challenges of living with CP says,

> I have average intelligence, but some people assume I'm mentally challenged just because of my physical limitations—especially my speech impairment. I feel if I could articulate my thoughts better, I would be accepted as the intelligent person that I am. . . . Writing has given me a voice I never had before and has helped me disprove various misconceptions the general public has concerning individuals with disabilities.[9]

Like Kayla, both children and adults with dysarthria must often endure impatient listeners who do not let them complete a spoken thought. Others write them off as "retarded" and refuse to interact at all. Before the age of computers few options for alternative means of communication were available. A person had to spell out or indicate his or her needs on letter boards or picture boards, which was extremely time-consuming. Today, it is possible for many with dysarthria and other motor speech difficulties to communicate more effectively through the use of computer-assisted devices and voice synthesizers.

Apraxia of Speech

Apraxia of speech, or verbal apraxia, is a motor speech disorder caused by damage to the parts of the brain related to speaking. People with verbal apraxia have trouble saying what they want to say correctly and consistently. They may have trouble with the rhythm and timing of speech, or they may say something completely different from what they intended, even making up words. Somewhat surprisingly, however, they may still be able to produce automatic phrases such as "How are you?" or "Fine, thank you" without any difficulty. Unlike dysarthria, verbal apraxia has nothing to do with a weakness or paralysis of the speech muscles. Apraxia may be exhibited as an articulation, fluency, or voice disorder, or a combination of the three. The severity can range from mild to severe.

Developmental Apraxia of Speech (DAS)

Developmental apraxia, or DAS, is one of two kinds of verbal apraxia. DAS (also sometimes called CAS for childhood apraxia of speech) occurs in children, is present from birth, and generally affects more boys than girls. As expected, children who suffer with this disorder do not babble as infants, and first words are delayed. But as they get older they may also have difficulty with long phrases and may appear to be searching for the words to express what they are thinking. Although children with DAS are usually able to understand language well, listeners are likely to have a difficult time understanding their speech.

Cause of DAS

The cause of DAS is not yet known. Scientists are divided in their opinions about whether DAS is a language disorder or a neurological disorder that affects the brain's ability to send the proper signals necessary for speech. In recent studies, however, brain imaging has not shown any evidence of specific brain lesions or differences from other children in brain structure. Instead, it has been observed that children with DAS often have family members who have a history of communication disorders or learning disabilities, which suggests a genetic cause.

Some research has indicated that the brain's natural ability to change its own structure (neuroplasticity) can help children with DAS create new learning pathways for the development of speech. Megan Hodge, an SLP who is researching the way

Developmental apraxia of speech can make the patient feel blindfolded, gagged, and unable to communicate.

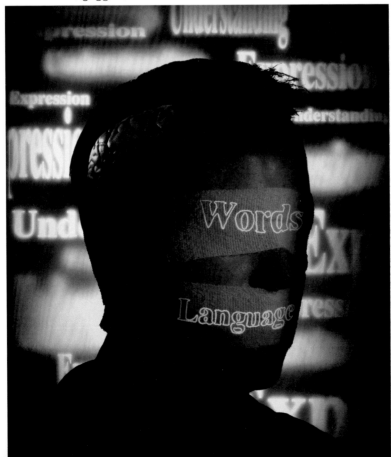

neuroplasticity affects speech development, is convinced early intervention is key. "A common report from parents is that their child with suspected CAS was a 'quiet' baby," she observes. "Children who are less communicative typically receive far fewer learning opportunities to 'practice' communicating when in fact, they need many more than other children do . . . from an early age we need to alter these babies' environments and multiply their opportunities to engage in experiences that promote speech learning."[10]

Speech disorders such as stuttering, lisps, DAS, and dysarthria frequently appear in early childhood. With time and therapy normal speech is sometimes possible. When it is not, children afflicted with severe speech disorders are more likely to adjust to the situation than adults even if they never learn to speak intelligibly.

Acquired Apraxia

Acquired apraxia of speech can affect a person of any age but typically occurs in adults and results in the loss or impairment of a person's existing ability to speak. It may be the result of a stroke, head injury, tumor, or other illness affecting the brain. Due to damage in the left frontal lobe of the brain, the ability to plan and coordinate the precise order of motor movements for speech is lost. Apraxia affects adults differently than children because language is already developed. The most common symptom in adults is difficulty in putting words and syllables together in the correct order. A person suffering from acquired apraxia is fully aware of his or her own speech errors and usually makes repeated attempts to correct them.

A conversation about a vacation to California with someone who has acquired apraxia might go something like this example found in a speech therapy textbook:

O-o-on . . . on . . . on our cavation, cavation, cacation . . . oh darn . . . vavation, oh, you know, to Ca-ca-caciporenia . . . no, Lacifacnia, vafacnia to Lacifacnion. . . . On our vacation to Vacafornia, no darn it . . . to Ca-caliborneo . . .

not bornia . . . fornia, Bornifornia . . . no, Ballifomeo, Bal-lifornee, Ballifornee, Californee, California. Phew, it was hard to say Cacaforneo. Oh darn.[11]

Although the formation of the word "California" was a strug-gle, this same individual may be able to say the word without hesitation at a different time. Afterward, it would not be a sur-prise to hear this same person say something like, "Wow, I sure had a tough time saying the word 'California' earlier."

Acquired apraxia of speech in adults sometimes corrects itself spontaneously. However, symptoms can be so severe the individual is left with virtually no speech at all. In such cases an alternative means of communication becomes necessary. This may include the use of simple hand gestures, sign lan-guage, electronic letter and picture boards, or a voice synthe-sizer. The type of communication device a person is able to use depends on the degree to which other parts of his or her body

Choosing the Right Speech Therapist

• Ask a pediatrician or family doctor to make a referral, or con-tact a teacher or local audiologist to ask for a recommendation.
• Look for someone who is certified by the American-Speech-Hearing Association (ASHA).
• Have a private consultation with the therapist you are consid-ering to see how you (or your child) will interact with them.
• Make sure the clinic or therapist you are considering uses a variety of therapies and an audiologist is available to check for hearing problems.
• Reevaluate the therapy and your (or your child's) progress of-ten. Do not be afraid to speak up if the therapy is not working.

are affected by apraxia, dysarthria, or some other disorder affecting muscle control.

Apraxia of speech rarely occurs alone. It is most often accompanied by dysarthria, aphasia (a language disorder), or both. At times it may be difficult to determine which of these conditions a sufferer may be exhibiting since all three tend to generate similar symptoms.

Spasmodic Dysphonia

In some cases the onset of an adult disorder has no specific event attached and appears relatively suddenly and mysteriously. Spasmodic dysphonia (SD) is one such mysterious voice disorder caused by involuntary movements or spasms of the vocal cords. This creates interruptions in the flow of speech and causes speech to be jerky, quivery, hoarse, tight, or have a groaning quality. Sometimes a person with spasmodic dysphonia has periods of near normal voice with intermittent periods of no voice (aphonia) and periods of poor vocal quality.

Spasmodic dysphonia is most common among women age thirty to fifty. According to the National Institute on Deafness and Other Communication Diseases, the exact cause of the disorder is not known. However, evidence does suggest it may be neurological and could be an inherited trait triggered by infections, stress, or injury. Spasmodic dysphonia has no cure, although several treatments are available, including the use of botulinum toxin (Botox) injections into one or both vocal chords to weaken the muscles that bring the vocal folds together. This leaves more room for breathing and usually improves voice quality. Unlike other treatments, Botox is not permanent. The injection must be repeated about every three months, which provides the opportunity to experiment with the placement and amount needed for best results.

Spasmodic dysphonia and several other speech disorders are common enough to be known by a specific label or name. In some cases the exact cause is still unknown. In addition to these disorders, however, many speech disorders are known by the conditions and diseases that cause them.

CHAPTER THREE

Conditions and Diseases That Cause Speech Disorders

Many physical conditions and diseases impair various bodily functions. Some of these functions are closely tied to the production of speech. The resulting speech disorders are characterized by the condition or disease that causes them.

Articulation Disorder Caused by Cleft Lip or Palate

Some speech disorders are directly related to a facial deformity known as a cleft lip or palate. A cleft lip is a visible gap or narrow opening on one or both sides of the upper lip that extend all the way to the base of the nose. A cleft palate, a gap or opening in the roof of the mouth called an isolated cleft, is only visible by examining the interior of the mouth. Clefts occur when the tissues of the mouth and lip do not form properly before birth.

During normal fetal development the tissue that will become the lip joins and fuses about five to six weeks after conception. The palate comes together and fuses at about seven weeks. Each year in the United States about sixty-eight hundred children are born with a cleft lip, a cleft palate, or both.

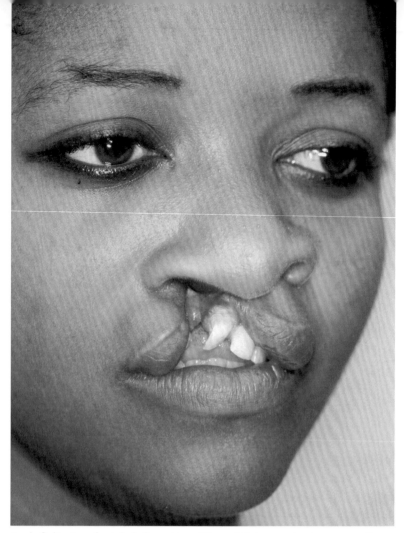

A cleft lip is a facial deformity with a visible gap in the upper lip that extends all the way to the base of the nose.

Challenges Associated with Clefts

Cleft palates and lips are not life threatening and, and in most cases, are not associated with any other birth defects. They are, however, a health problem. Newborns with these deformities usually have trouble feeding because they cannot create enough suction to pull on the nipple of a bottle or breast. A child with an unrepaired cleft may be prone to ear infections because the Eustachian tubes do not drain fluid from the middle ear to the throat properly. Teeth may be misaligned, causing dental problems. These factors also affect speech development and can lead to severe articulation disorders.

Healing Smiles and Transforming Lives

In 1982 plastic surgeon William P. Magee Jr. and his wife, Kathleen, a nurse, traveled to the Philippines with a group of medical volunteers to repair cleft lips and palates of the local children. Although they helped many people, the volunteers were forced to turn away hundreds more who were ravaged by facial deformities. The Magees quickly realized a program was needed that would provide medical treatment and training in countries around the world. Returning home to the United States they established Operation Smile.

Since its inception in 1982 Operation Smile has treated more than 130,000 children and young adults with facial deformities. They have worked in fifty-one countries worldwide providing free surgeries, training local medical professionals, and leaving behind crucial medical equipment to allow their work to continue long after they are gone.

In November 2007 Operation Smile celebrated its twenty-fifth anniversary with the World Journey of Smiles. During this initiative Operation Smile volunteers visited twenty-five different countries on forty simultaneous missions. When it was over, 4,086 children had been given new smiles and a new lease on life.

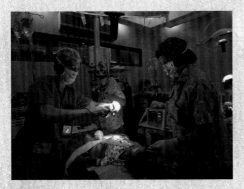

Operation Smile volunteer surgeons prepare to perform cleft palate corrective surgery on a child in the Philippines. In more than twenty-five years, the organization has treated over 130,000 children for facial deformities.

Cleft Palate Speech

A cleft palate produces speech that is nasal in quality and can be hard to understand. Forming sounds for letters such as "t," "k," "s," "sh," "d," and "x" is difficult because these and other consonants require contact between the palate and tongue. A cleft palate has less tissue for the tongue to touch. Vowels may sound especially nasal because they are produced inside the mouth on a controlled breath. People with an unrepaired cleft are unable to produce these sounds properly because air escapes through the nose. They do not have the ability to "hold their breath" or control the release of a breath.

It usually takes many surgeries over a number of years to fully correct a cleft lip and palate. Ongoing speech therapy during these years can help a person born with this defect to achieve normal speech.

Gina Butchin, an adult who was born with a bilateral (on both sides of the mouth) complete cleft lip and palate, underwent multiple surgeries as a child to repair the damage caused by the clefts. She remembers being "made fun of for having scars on my face and for talking funny, but I was not teased any more than the fat kid or the kid with the glasses. . . . My nose was flat, my scars were bad, my voice was difficult to understand at times, and yet I can honestly say I had a pretty normal childhood." Additional surgeries as an adult allowed Gina to improve her appearance, the quality of her voice, and achieve great personal growth. "At 40 years old," she says, "I can finally say that my surgeries are complete. I could not be happier with the way that I look and the way that I feel."[12]

People Affected by Clefts

A cleft is the most common major birth defect in the United States. Boys are more likely than girls to be born with cleft lips, but girls are more likely to have cleft palates. More common among Asians, Latinos, and Native Americans, clefts occur once in about seven hundred to one thousand births.

In today's age of highly specialized diagnostic equipment, cleft palates are rarely a surprise. Prenatal ultrasounds can detect the presence of a cleft before birth. If the defect escapes detection, it is easily identified at birth. In the United States resources are available to repair the damages, and the prognosis for normal speech and appearance is very good. Children born with clefts in developing countries are not so lucky. They are likely to suffer the physical and emotional effects of the defect for their entire lifetime.

Causes of Cleft Palate

Although the cause of clefts is unknown, doctors believe a combination of factors may be involved. Cleft palates seem to occur more often in children whose siblings or parents have a cleft or who have a history of clefts in their families. This indicates that the problem may be genetic. In addition, researchers have determined that women who smoke, drink alcohol, take certain medications or illicit drugs, or who are exposed to some viruses when pregnant may give birth to a baby with a cleft. They also speculate that certain nutritional deficiencies in the mother, such as a lack of folate, may be at fault. In these cases, if a gene for clefts is present, one or more of these factors may trigger the actual cleft.

Dysarthria Associated with Cerebral Palsy

Cerebral palsy is a group of disorders that affect two to three children out of every thousand in the United States. CP is usually the result of brain injury or damage occurring before, during, or just after birth. It affects both boys and girls of all ethnic groups. Individuals with CP have trouble controlling movement and maintaining balance. The severity depends on the amount of damage and to which areas of the brain.

About two-thirds of people with CP have impaired speech or language due to dysarthria. The type of speech problem depends largely on the type and extent of the brain injury.

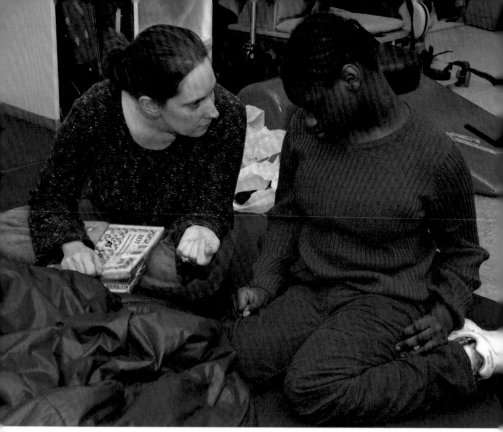

About two-thirds of people with cerebral palsy have impaired speech or language due to dysarthria.

Voice Disorders

Disorders related to voice are often temporary or, at the very least, treatable. In rare cases, however, a voice disorder makes communication difficult. Some people have an extremely high voice range (called puberphonia), a monotone, or an extremely low voice range (called dysphonia) due to the length and tension of the vocal folds. The speech of these individuals is startling at best. At times it can be annoying to listeners. The tension this creates between the speaker and the listener can cause many of the same kinds of psychological responses in the speaker as experienced by stutterers or cleft palate speakers.

Speech therapy can often help those suffering with a voice disorder, but only when the cause is physical. The effectiveness of the therapy is limited by the anatomy of the voice mechanism. In some cases, however, voice disorders are a symptom of a psychological disorder. If no physical reason for the symptoms is apparent, psychiatric treatment may be in order.

Voice Disorders Associated with Vocal Abuse

Screaming too loudly at a ball game, talking over noisy machinery, or singing for hours at a time are all examples of what SLPs call vocal abuse. Behaviors such as these may result in a temporary hoarseness or laryngitis—the mildest forms of a voice disorder. Vocal abuse that is not corrected, however, can lead to the formation of vocal nodules.

When operating normally, the vocal folds open and close in cycles to control the flow of air from the lungs and produce the sounds of speech. Vocal nodules are growths on the vocal folds that affect the quality of a person's speech. Growths on one or both vocal folds can keep them from functioning properly and create gaps that allow air to escape at the wrong time.

A person who develops nodules may sound hoarse, experience an inability to reach high or low tones, and have frequent unintended stops in the flow of speech. In addition, vocal nodules often result in a sore throat. This creates particular problems for those who depend on their voice to earn their living, especially speakers and singers.

Who Gets Vocal Nodules?

Vocal nodules are most common among women between the ages of twenty and fifty, but they can be a problem for anyone who uses his or her voice for long hours or who needs to speak loudly. This includes teachers, singers, auctioneers, lecturers, and members of the clergy. Early in their formation the nodules are soft and can be treated by simply resting the voice—that is, by not talking. If left untreated or if the vocal abuse continues, however, the nodules can become hard and fibrous, like a callus. When this happens surgery may be required to remove them. Once they are removed voice therapy is needed to train the person to use the voice differently. While the surgery is considered routine, it can be risky for someone like a professional singer.

In 1997 Julie Andrews, an actress and singer perhaps best known for her roles in *Mary Poppins* and *The Sound of Music*, underwent surgery to remove a noncancerous nodule on one vocal fold. As a result of her surgery the actress experienced permanent hoarseness and a greatly diminished range from what had been an impressive four octaves. Today, while she works to regain the singing voice she once had, her doctors tell her there is not much hope the damage can be repaired. Sadly, Julie says, "Not to sing with an orchestra or not to be able to communicate through my voice—which I've done all my life—and not to be able to phrase lyrics and give people that kind of joy is totally devastating."[13]

This illustration shows a polyp, or nodule, in beige, on a vocal chord.

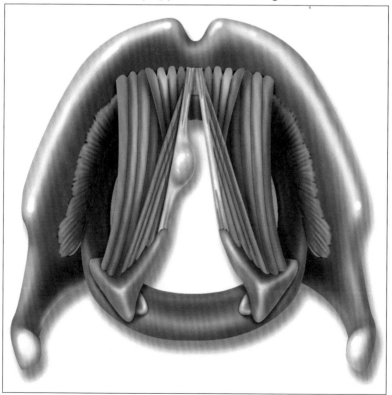

Perhaps due to experiences like Andrews', many people are becoming more conscientious about practicing what speech therapists call "good vocal hygiene." It is said that singer Celine Dion, for example, is careful to rest her voice regularly. She avoids situations that require shouting or screaming and limits her singing time in order to preserve her voice.

Singer Mariah Carey has already learned her lesson the hard way. A bout with vocal nodules has taught her to conserve her voice by taking a two-day vocal rest before a concert and communicating only by writing notes. She makes sure she gets plenty of rest, too, noting that sleep deprivation can interfere with her ability to hit the high notes.

Avoiding Vocal Nodules

As a rule vocal nodules are avoidable. Good vocal hygiene can help a person maintain voice quality well into their later years. Rest is a key component along with drinking plenty of water to keep the voice hydrated. Alcohol, caffeine, smoking, and the vocal extremes of shouting and whispering can all have a negative effect and should be avoided.

Other Disorders That Harm Vocal Folds

Several other conditions similar to vocal nodules can also damage the vocal folds. Vocal polyps (fluid filled lesions similar to blisters) and chronic laryngitis can interfere with vocal quality in much the same way as vocal nodules. Both of these conditions are generally caused by vocal abuse, although smoking, alcohol, or allergies can be a factor as well. In addition, contact ulcers, painful ulcers on both vocal cords caused by gastric reflux or habitual binging and purging (a symptom of bulimia), can produce the same symptoms.

Aside from the injuries and strokes that can happen at any age, a number of diseases can strike adults as they advance in years. Several of these diseases can have a devastating impact on the ability to speak normally.

Parkinson's Disease

Parkinson's disease is the second most common neurogenic disorder, occurring in about 1 percent of the population over age sixty. People of all ethnic origins can be affected, but men are slightly more likely to develop the disease than women. Due to damage of the central or peripheral nervous system, Parkinson's can create a whole host of symptoms. The cause of Parkinson's is still largely unknown.

About 89 percent of individuals with Parkinson's suffer from motor speech disorders such as dysarthria or apraxia as a result of damage to the brain and nervous system caused by their disease. Even though Parkinson's patients are aware of their diminished voice capacity, it may be that other symptoms of their disease are more alarming and therefore more likely to be the focus of any therapy. As a result few Parkinson's patients pursue speech therapy.

Huntington's Disease

Another neurological disease that can affect speech is Huntington's disease. Huntington's is a fatal brain disorder that causes certain brain cells to waste away. It progressively robs a person of the ability to control normal muscular movement and causes a decline in mental function until the person is in full dementia.

Huntington's affects about 5 out of 100,000 people. Symptoms may appear as early as age 35, but onset usually occurs in the late 40s and progresses unrelentingly for the next 15 to 20 years. Because an individual's cognitive and motor abilities are impaired, Huntington's hampers both the thought process related to speaking and the movements necessary to carry it out. The disease is an inherited condition caused by a single defective gene. Anyone born with the gene will eventually develop Huntington's if they live long enough.

Amyotrophic Lateral Sclerosis

Like Huntington's, amyotrophic lateral sclerosis, or ALS, is a progressive, fatal disease that strikes older adults. With a

Michael J. Fox Foundation

Following in the footsteps of Jerry Lewis and his efforts to promote awareness and research for muscular dystrophy, actor Michael J. Fox has chosen to lend his celebrity star power to fighting a disease, too—in this case Parkinson's disease. The difference is that Fox himself suffers from the disease.

First diagnosed in 1991, Fox did not reveal his condition until 1998. Following his retirement from the sitcom *Spin City* in January 2000, he launched the Michael J. Fox Foundation for Parkinson's Research. The foundation is dedicated to finding a cure for Parkinson's within the next ten years.

Since its inception the Michael J. Fox Foundation has become the largest private funder of medical research related to Parkinson's in the United States. The foundation awards grants to ensure that the most promising research avenues are properly funded and explored in the hope of finding new therapies and eventually a cure. As of 2009, the foundation has funded more than $142 million in research directly or through partnerships.

Michael J. Fox's foundation has become the largest private funder of medical research into Parkinson's disease in the United States.

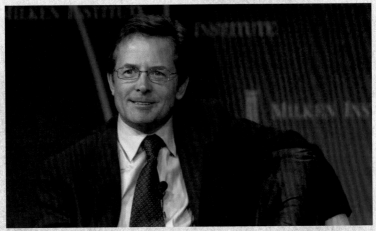

survival rate of only three to five years, ALS tends to progress much more rapidly than Huntington's. ALS attacks the nerve cells responsible for controlling voluntary muscles. Eventually patients lose strength and the ability to move their arms, legs, and body.

ALS also produces dysarthria and/or apraxia, causing speech to be unpredictable and difficult to understand. This is often accompanied by dysphagia, an inability to swallow properly. By the time the muscles of the diaphragm and chest wall fail, patients lose the ability to breathe on their own. Because the disease does not affect cognitive abilities, ALS patients are aware of their progressive loss of function and often become anxious and depressed about their condition.

The cause of ALS is not entirely understood. About 5 to 10 percent of cases are inherited, but the other 90 to 95 percent occur at random. As many as 200,000 Americans have ALS, and an estimated 5,000 new cases are diagnosed in the United States each year. The disease is almost two times more common in men than women.

Cancer

Cancer can also affect speech. Always frightening, cancer can be especially devastating to those who develop the disease in the area of the mouth, tongue, or throat. This is due to the rather extreme and often highly visible measures that must be taken to treat cancer in these locations.

Oral cancer includes cancers of the mouth, tongue, back portions of the throat (pharynx), and larynx. Many of these cancers begin in the mouth and can spread quickly if left untreated. Typically oral cancer occurs after age forty and is twice as common in men as women. Those who use tobacco and/or drink alcohol heavily greatly increase their risk of developing the disease. Currently in the United States, about thirty-four thousand people are affected by some form of oral cancer.

Because oral cancer affects the muscles and tissues associated with speech, an individual's voice quality and/or ability to articulate clearly can be hampered by both the cancer and

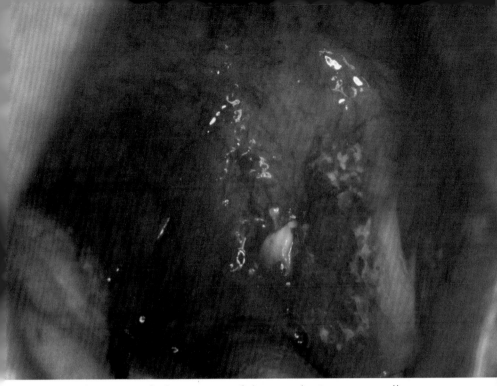

Oral cancer includes cancers of the mouth. Cancerous cells are shown in white.

the efforts to eradicate it. The treatments necessary for later stages generally involve surgery along with radiation and/or chemotherapy. Sometimes the removal of tissues or organs that are necessary for speech may require a survivor to learn an entirely new way of speaking.

Laryngectomy

Cancer of the throat and/or larynx sometimes requires the removal of the entire larynx. This requires repositioning the trachea to allow the patient to breathe through a hole in the throat called a stoma. Once the larynx is gone, the source of the individual's voice is also gone, and he or she must learn an alternate method of producing the sounds necessary for speech. For some, this means using an electronic device called an electrolarynx. This allows the person to have a voice, of sorts, which has a robotlike quality.

Many electrolarynx users can testify to being mistaken for robots or computers, especially on the phone. One man tells of answering the phone and being asked by the caller if "there was a human being there" he could speak with. The caller was genuinely surprised to find he was already talking with one.

Another method of producing voice sounds is esophageal speech. This requires individuals to use their esophagus as a source of vibrations to produce sounds. Essentially, they speak on "burps" in the absence of vocal folds. The idea may seem funny at first, since many people often demonstrate this ability as a joke. However, day-to-day speech done in this manner is very tiresome and certainly no joke.

Deaf and Hard of Hearing Speech

As might be expected, the inability to hear the sounds of speech makes it particularly difficult to learn to produce them. Although not an impossible task, most deaf people never learn to speak clearly. For someone who has been deaf from birth, learning to speak plainly is considered a tremendous accomplishment. Those who are not deaf but hard of hearing often struggle to master the articulation of sounds they cannot hear clearly. Because a deaf or hard of hearing person is unable to monitor pitch and loudness, his or her speech tends to have a monotone quality to it at a pitch that seems a bit unnatural.

As many as 28.6 million Americans have some degree of hearing loss. This number might actually be much larger, considering a 2004 report that suggests nearly half of the U.S. baby boomer generation (adults born from 1945 to 1959) are also affected by hearing loss. In children, 1 in 1,000 is born deaf while another 83 have an "educationally significant" hearing loss. This is any hearing loss that impacts an individual's ability to learn or the methods that must be used to educate them. No matter what the age of onset, however, hearing loss can produce a wide range of psychological, social, and emotional consequences. Difficulty in acquiring or producing understandable speech is just one of them.

Children who are born with a hearing loss usually exhibit speech difficulties early on. Many people who are hard of hearing are able to hear vowel sounds better than consonants.

Without the consonants, however, the understanding of speech is lost. For children learning to talk, this missing information makes the task much more difficult. Early speech therapy intervention is extremely important.

A hearing loss in adults tends to have a more emotional effect than it does in children. Adults already know how to talk, but a hearing loss in later years often means the individual is no longer able to participate in certain activities with the same success as they did in the past. Adults who experience a hearing loss are often unable to enjoy private conversations, talk on the phone, participate in meetings, or keep up with the flow of conversation in large gatherings. The frustration and anger they experience can eventually lead to depression and a tendency to withdraw from social contact.

Children born with hearing loss need early speech therapy so they will not fall behind in school.

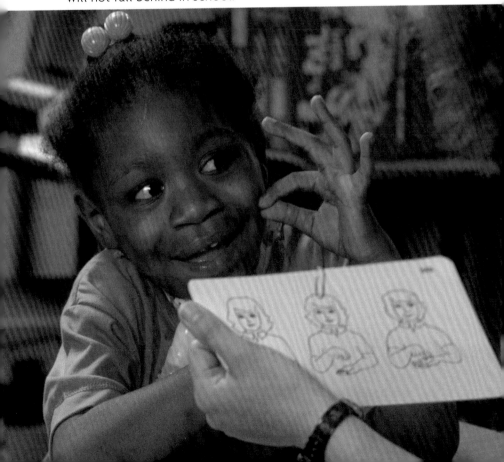

In general, speech disorders can be devastating for adults. Many of the diseases and injuries that cause the disorders are debilitating or even fatal. While speech therapy can benefit some, many adults are never able to completely regain the speech they have lost, and they find it difficult to adjust to life without the ability to communicate as they once did. The emotional toll is sometimes as great as the injury or illness that caused the speech disorder in the first place.

CHAPTER FOUR

Living with a Speech Disorder

Speech and communication problems that are not corrected by time or therapy can become a daily struggle for those who must live with them. Any speech disorder has the potential to affect many areas of a person's life. And, while some are able to master their disorder, others find themselves struggling to cope.

Many people who live with a speech disorder suffer from depression due to a poor self-image. They are afraid to meet new people because they believe they will not be taken seriously or, even worse, that they will be openly ridiculed. As a result they often feel socially inept. Facing the problem by deliberately seeking out opportunities to talk with others or seeking help through speech therapy takes a tremendous amount of courage. Those who cannot summon this courage often find themselves bound by their own regrets and anxieties.

Some people, however, refuse to allow their speech disorder to dictate their behavior. Instead, they choose to face their fears head-on. In doing this, many have discovered that what they thought was so terrible is actually a catalyst for developing character and perseverance. In the end, they realize that the disorder itself is never the problem—the way a person deals with and responds to it is what matters.

Living with a Lisp

Although a lisp is generally considered correctable, many people manage to make it into their adult years without ever having dealt with the issue. What did not seem to be such a big deal when they were young suddenly begins to have a negative impact on their education, work, or social life. Working to correct the disorder is much more difficult as an adult than as a child.

A twenty-three-year-old education student found this out when she began student teaching. Although she always had a lisp, she was never really bothered by it until it began to affect

Children with speech disorders can suffer from depression because they are often shunned or openly ridiculed.

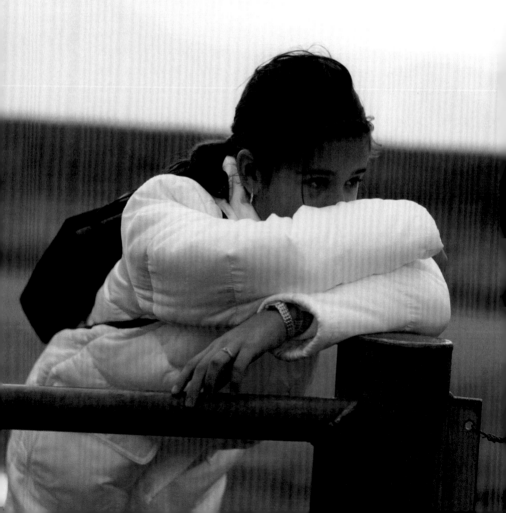

her work. As she began practice teaching, the kids made comments and often imitated her, much to her dismay. The last straw came when a parent told her supervising teacher that her speech was not a good example for the children. "I am so sick of the comments," she says. "I actually cried when it happened."[14]

Although this young woman did not pay much attention to her lisp until it began to affect her career, many others struggle with it from the beginning. In an Internet video post sixteen-year-old Loki notes,

> Having a lisp is not an easy thing to overcome. . . . Anybody who doesn't have a lisp and doesn't know the torture that these people who have lisps and stuff like that have to go through every day—with the mechanics of speech and the people making fun of you—put that together—and you have to think about what you have to say before you say the words—put those, put all three of that together, combine them in a pot, and then see how you would feel if you had a lisp. . . . It's a sad thing to have a lisp.[15]

Early intervention is the best approach for any speech disorder. Sometimes waiting until adolescence or adulthood can lead to the development of poor social skills. People who are embarrassed by their speech often fail to make eye contact when they speak to others, have poor posture, and fail to smile when speaking. Not only do these behaviors fail to "win friends and influence people," but they may also impede educational or professional development.

Living with Stuttering

The social stigma associated with lisping can be even worse for those who stutter. Few people with normal speech have the patience and sensitivity to allow a stutterer to finish a thought. Some try to finish the sentence in an effort to help, while others simply walk away in disgust, somehow convinced that stuttering signals a lack of intelligence. The more a stutterer is

Famous People with Speech Disorders

Speech disorders do not have to be a barrier to achievement. Many famous people have made great accomplishments while dealing with various types of speech difficulties:

Stutter: Aristotle, Winston Churchill, Samuel Jackson, James Earl Jones, Julia Roberts, Jeremiah Taylor, Mel Tillis, Bruce Willis, Tiger Woods

Lisp: Humphrey Bogart, Winston Churchill, Thomas Jefferson, Elton John, Barbara Walters

Vocal nodules: Mariah Carey, Whitney Houston, Elton John, Justin Timberlake

Cleft lip: Jesse Jackson, Peyton Manning, Cheech Marin, King Tutankhamen

Winston Churchill speaks before the U.S. Congress in 1952. A stutterer, he became one of the great speakers of the twentieth century.

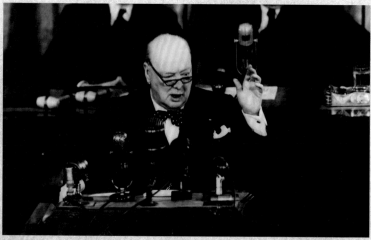

exposed to this sort of behavior, the more he or she is inclined to withdraw.

Walter H. Manning, a University of Memphis professor, remembers a time when he avoided speaking at all costs. "For many years stuttering was shameful, painful and embarrassing—something to be denied and certainly hidden." But after some intensive therapy during his days at Penn State University, Manning began to see himself and his stuttering in a different light. "It was exciting to understand that I wasn't the problem," he says. "The problem was stuttering—and I had some choices about how I might respond and change my relationship with stuttering."[16] His discovery allowed him to finally view his stuttering as a gift—one that has enabled him to enter an interesting field of study and experience what he considers an exciting career. Not every stutterer has such a positive attitude.

A photographer with California's *Orange County Register*, Ken Steinhardt, is a severe stutterer. Although he has periods of fluency, he calls them "temporary." "I refer to my fluency as temporary," he writes, "because I can't count on it. I can count on my stuttering. Like all stutterers, I sing with fluency." Over the years Ken struggled to come to terms with his stuttering, even participating (with some success) in a drug trial in 2006. In spite of his guarded optimism about the future of drug therapy he notes, "After 41 years as a severe stutterer, from all the speech therapy I went through—and I went through a lot—I have come to accept the fact that there is no cure for stuttering. . . . Fluency is earned through work. Talking about it, and writing, helps. Both are part of my therapy."[17]

Most people who stutter eventually reach a point where they accept their condition and resolve to move on in spite of it. Stuttering need not stand in the way of success, as scores of people have discovered. Pamela Mertz has achieved a new freedom in her life by refusing to allow her stuttering to keep her silent. She and other stutterers have learned a valuable secret—no one is defined by their stuttering unless they allow themselves to be.

Living with a Cleft Lip or Palate

Many stutterers discover that the journey they must travel through life, although often painful, eventually makes them stronger. Those who are born with a cleft lip or palate frequently arrive at the same conclusion—but the pain of their journey can be more than just emotional.

A cleft palate or lip is a repairable birth defect requiring multiple surgeries. It is not uncommon for a person to have ten to twenty surgeries or more over the course of his or her lifetime. The surgeries usually begin just a few months after birth and continue until the patient is well into adulthood. The surgeries can be painful, and extensive dental work is often required as well. Rose Senerchia, a woman now in her forties, endured approximately twenty-five surgeries by the time she was twenty-two. "Having one surgery after another when you are young is not easy," she says. "It's very scary. But it has made me a stronger person."[18]

Many others with clefts tend to agree. Growing up with facial scars and talking differently usually means being a target for bullies. Learning how to handle bullies is not pleasant, but facing the problem head-on leads to greater maturity and develops a "can do" attitude. Kendall Tullis, now a young adult, recalls how she was teased as a child. "When I was little, I used to think if I just ignored people who picked on me, they would stop. But I soon realized that sometimes I could not just go on letting people belittle me, so I faced the bullies," she says. "Having a cleft palate sometimes makes you have to act older than you really are because you have experienced more than most people will in their lifetime."[19]

Enduring a cleft lip or palate is not easy, but surprisingly, many who have say they would not change a thing. They say that dealing with the challenges associated with a cleft develops character. Some, like Rose, recognize that "life is not about all the pain and heartaches, but what you make out of it all. Yes, it would be wonderful to look like everyone else. But then I wonder what kind of person I would be and I realize that I would not be me."[20] Claire Crawford, a Mississippi

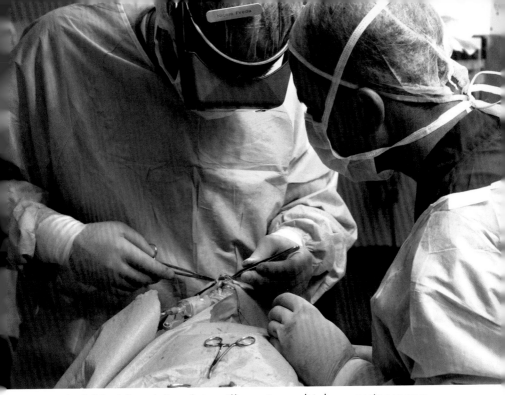

A child with a cleft palate will require multiple surgeries over a period of time.

woman born with a cleft lip and palate, agrees. "Having a cleft is not a tragedy that will be suffered forever," she says, "but an obstacle in life that can be overcome. My cleft is a part of me, not what defines me."[21]

Lisps, stuttering, and clefts can interfere with speech at an early age, before or just as a child is acquiring language skills. Other disorders appear postlingually and can present a whole different set of frustrations.

Living with Dysarthria

People who suffer with CP, Parkinson's, and other diseases that affect muscle strength and control are victims of dysarthria. They struggle with an increased danger of choking, diminished voice quality, and difficulty finding words and formulating ideas. Their speech may be slurred, the tone or pitch may change, or, because they lack the strength to keep it going, their voice may trail off to a whisper. People suffering with dysarthria may feel as though they are shouting even though

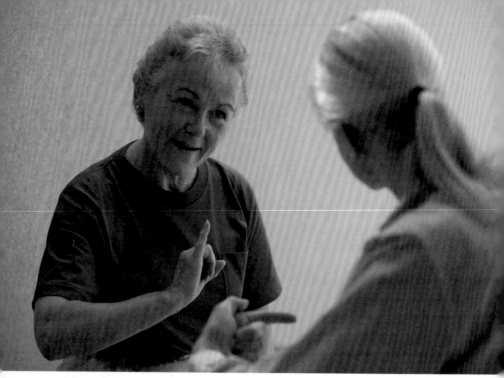

Although dysarthria has no cure, speech therapy and sign language can help patients to express themselves.

their listeners can barely hear them. Many report difficulties in staying on task—frequently losing their train of thought in the process of trying to verbalize it.

For those who attempt conversation, additional obstacles exist. Not only are their own bodies working against them but they must often endure rude or overly helpful listeners. Dysarthria victims say talking is hard work—made harder by the embarrassment of stares or irritation when they do not finish a thought quickly enough. Participating in even the shortest exchange becomes so difficult that many opt to become passive listeners rather than put forth the effort to engage in conversation. Some become completely withdrawn, avoiding any situations that require talking.

A person with dysarthria may have such slurred speech that even close friends and family do not understand him or her. Listeners, trying to be polite, often pretend to understand rather than ask the speaker to repeat something for the third or fourth time. A speaker who recognizes such pretense may feel that the listeners do not care about what he or she was trying to say. Even people who have lived together for many years can have trouble communicating due to the effects of dysarthria. The frustration level for both the speaker and listeners can be quite high.

Although dysarthria cannot be cured, speech therapy can help. Those who receive therapy are able to learn alternative methods for using their voice. Those who use computers find e-mail a great way to say what they want to say because they can spend as long as they like composing their thoughts. Sign language, gestures, and communication boards are other alternatives for self-expression. People with dysarthria want others to know how hard they are working to communicate. Listeners who maintain a positive and patient attitude do much to bolster such speakers' confidence and self-esteem.

Living with a Voice Disorder

Having a voice that calls attention to the speaker can be a good thing—for a professional speaker or singer. If attention is paid because a person's voice sounds "funny," the speaker may feel embarrassed or unhappy. In addition, voice disorders sometimes cause changes that take away a speaker's normal voice. In these situations people often despair about losing the sound of his or her "own voice."

Elizabeth Bachini clearly remembers the last time she enjoyed having a normal voice. During a 2004 Thanksgiving celebration she entertained her family with her singing while her father played the piano. That winter she developed a persistent sore throat accompanied by a hoarse, scratchy voice. By mid-2005 she had been diagnosed with spasmodic dysphonia.

Refusing to give in to her disorder, Elizabeth has struggled through job interviews, won the respect of her colleagues, and pursued her professional goals—all in spite of her vocal imperfections. No longer able to sing or speak clearly, the loss of her normal voice has been both a physical and mental challenge.

Reflecting on her voice difficulties, Elizabeth says, "I have left classes humiliated by my peers' winces at the sound of my voice; and I have walked back in, raised my hand, and participated anyway." Her singing ability is sorely missed. "Often, I will hear a great song and open my mouth to sing, and then abruptly realize I cannot project sound as I once did," she notes. "I suppose that is the small sacrifice I will have to make for finding a strength I did not know existed within me . . . one which sustains me and pushes me ever forward."[22]

Although Elizabeth may never find her normal voice again, many who suffer with voice disorders can benefit from education about the proper vocal techniques. Melissa Fitzpatrick, a nurse and vice president of a medical technologies firm, began experiencing voice problems in 2006. As a motivational speaker and the coach for her son's basketball team, Melissa's voice was getting quite the workout. After hearing her talk in Virginia, an SLP in the audience recognized the voice characteristics of damaged vocal chords. At the SLPs suggestion Melissa sought medical help and soon after was diagnosed with noncancerous lesions on one vocal fold.

Opting for therapy rather than surgery, Melissa has learned to use her voice without straining it. "I'm much more careful about my screaming, cheering and acting like a nut," she says. "These are good strategies for moms who are at home yelling at kids, hailing a cab—things you don't realize put a strain and stress on vocal cords. You only get two of them."[23] Due to her work with an SLP, Melissa has been able to reduce the size of the lesions, keep them from spreading, and restore her normal voice.

Living as a Laryngectomee

Because no amount of therapy will get rid of cancer, surgery is often the only option. Waking up after surgery to remove the larynx, patients face confusing and dramatic changes. Laryngectomees, people who have had their larynx (voice box) removed, breathe through a hole in the throat called a stoma. Without any vocal folds to produce voice, laryngectomees must learn a completely new way of talking.

Laryngectomy patients usually begin learning to talk again with the aid of an electrolarynx. These electronic devices pro-

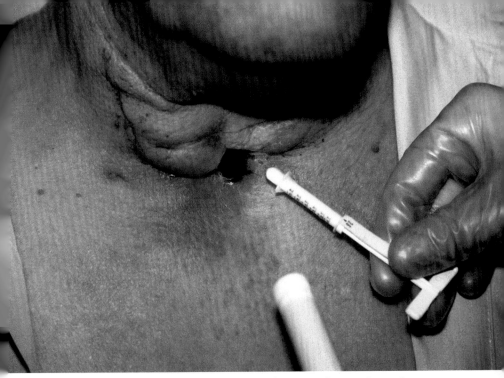

A speech therapist inserts a voice valve into the trachea of a laryngectomee to give him the ability to speak electronically.

vide the vibrations necessary for sounds that had previously originated in the vocal folds. Laryngectomees soon learn their new "voice" takes some getting used to.

Laryngectomee Patsy Armstrong tells of coming home to find a message on the answering machine. She could tell it was from a "lary" but was unable to understand any part of the message except her husband's name. When she played it for her husband, she was shocked to discover that it was a message she herself had left for him.

Fellow laryngectomee, Michael Csapo, relates a story about arguing with a telemarketer on the phone. Angry that he had been unable to make his point he fumed to his wife that "arguing with those people is just a waste of breath."[24] His wife was quick to point out his error. "You mean arguing with them is a waste of batteries, don't you?"[25]

Laryngectomees have several options when it comes to regaining their speech. Other than the electorlarynx, a person may use esophageal speech (which is very difficult to learn) or a tracheoesophageal puncture and prosthesis. A tracheoesophageal puncture is a small hole made through the wall of the trachea into the esophagus. Later, a prosthesis is inserted into the hole, allowing exhaled air to travel through the esophagus. By covering the stoma with a special valve, or simply with a thumb, a laryngectomee can "talk" on the vibrations of the esophageal walls. Occasionally laryngectomees are asked if they have a microphone in their thumb or what they are hiding under it.

In spite of their convenience, mishaps with tracheal prostheses are not uncommon. C.W. Moreland remembers a time when he accidently pushed his prosthesis into his esophagus and promptly swallowed it. A visit to the ear, nose, and throat doctor assured him that he had no need to worry since the object would pass in time. Moreland wrote about the incident as an encouragement to other laryngectomees. "I was so concerned with what might happen prior to it passing that I was afraid to pass gas for fear of not knowing what it would say!"[26]

Most people who have had a laryngectomy are able to regain a form of speech they are comfortable with. However, any option they choose takes some getting used to as well as practice in order to be understood.

Learning a new way to talk is just one of the challenges associated with the removal of the voice box. Basic procedures for the care of the stoma, recovery from the surgery itself, and lifestyle changes also must be dealt with. Web Whispers is an international Internet support group that provides information and support for members of this rather unique club. Begun in 1996, Web Whispers is now the largest support group for laryngectomees, offering advice and education to those who need it from those who have experienced it.

Living with a Hearing Impairment

Not being able to hear the sounds of speech presents special challenges to those who live with a hearing impairment. Holly, a twenty-nine-year-old deaf adult, is well educated and has achieved a certain level of success in her job. She lives on her

Rockin' and Rollin' After a Stroke

Dick Clark is an American radio and television personality and game show host. Often called "America's Oldest Teenager" for his youthful appearance, Clark gained a place in pop culture history as the host of *American Bandstand* and the annual *Dick Clark's New Year's Rockin' Eve* party in Times Square, New York.

In early December 2004 Clark suffered a stroke and was unable to attend the 2005 New Year's celebration for the first time in thirty-three years. After an intense year of learning to walk and talk again, Clark returned to welcome 2006 on December 31, 2005, cohosting with *American Idol* host Ryan Seacrest. Although his speech was slurred and somewhat muffled, he managed a quick pace and was generally understandable. It was clear Clark had worked hard to return to an event he "wouldn't miss for the world."

Clark has cohosted each New Year's party since 2005, his speech and mobility improving with each year. He plans to continue as the show's cohost through 2010 to ring in 2011. Stroke survivors across America have been encouraged by his example, praising him as an inspiration.

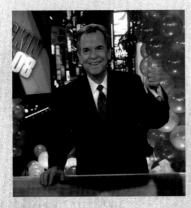

Dick Clark returned to host his TV show *New Year's Rockin' Eve* in 2005 after recovering from a stroke and learning to walk and talk again.

own, supports herself, and operates well in both the "hearing world" and that of the deaf. Her primary language, however, is American Sign Language (ASL). For Holly, English is a second language—one she struggles with in much the same way other nonnative speakers do. While she has some speech, producing it takes a lot of effort on her part and is generally not understood by people outside her family. She is most comfortable conversing in her "native language," ASL.

In spite of Holly's speech limitations, she does not see herself as "handicapped." Because she has never heard, she does not miss it. In many ways she has been able to adjust to her situation better than someone who is simply hard of hearing or who experiences hearing loss after years of normal hearing.

For those who are hard of hearing but not profoundly deaf, the acquisition of speech is a process filled with trial and error. Day-to-day living is quite different. Devon, a communications disorders major in college, understands this firsthand since he grew up in a home with a hard of hearing parent. "I had to repeat myself most of the time while talking to her [his mother]," he explains. "I had to speak clearly, and most of all, I could not cover my mouth. My mother reads lips."[27] Although Devon's mother has learned to speak, participating in any conversation takes more effort on her part than it might for someone with normal hearing.

Most people give little thought to being able to say whatever is on their mind. Ironically, those who struggle with speech disorders sometimes think of nothing else. Some, through great effort, are able to overcome their particular speech difficulty and return to normal speech. Others must learn to embrace a new way of communicating in order to be heard. No matter how communication is reestablished, living with a speech disorder presents a unique challenge. It takes a strong will and the help of a speech professional to overcome the obstacles that come with a speech disorder.

CHAPTER FIVE

Diagnosis and Treatment of Speech Disorders

The treatment of a speech disorder almost always involves speech therapy. SLPs work with a wide variety of both speech and language disorders in an effort to help clients achieve or return to normal speech. Some experience more success than others.

How Effective Is Speech Therapy?

Because speech pathology is a relatively new field, some still debate the effectiveness of speech therapy. In the mid-1990s, speech pathologist and therapist Virginia Pearson authored a review of the literature in which she cautioned, "There is a need for better information about effectiveness in many areas of speech and language therapists' work" along with a need for additional information on "the most efficient and effective way of delivering a speech and language therapy service."[28]

Not long afterward, British SLP Pam Enderby and author Joyce Emerson speculated that the difficulty in measuring the effectiveness of speech therapy is due to the wide variety of therapy methods being used. In addition, these methods are being applied to an extremely wide range of communication

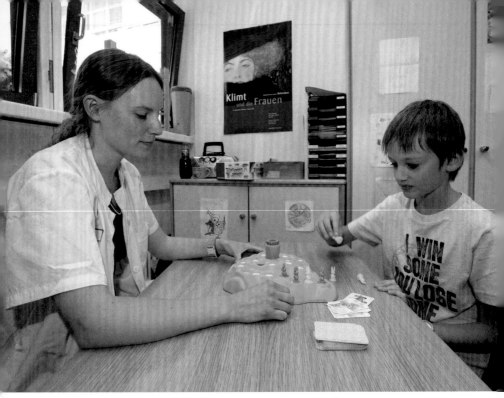

A speech therapist and a child play a game in a therapy session. There are many different ideas about how to treat speech disorders.

disorders. They point out that the goals of therapy are usually broader than just improving speech or language and might include "providing alternative methods to communicate, improving interaction strategies [overall communication skills], and advising patients and relatives." They believe that as therapy techniques and objectives are refined and become more clearly defined, "research done as recently as a decade ago may look simplistic and inappropriate,"[29] and that the overall effectiveness of therapy techniques will improve as more is learned about this field of study.

It appears, then, that researching individual speech therapies enough to prove which are successful and which are not in strictly scientific terms will take time. In the meantime, many SLPs believe the effectiveness of the services they provide is readily apparent. They point to cases such as Andrew, who was diagnosed with a developmental speech disorder as a three-year-old. Doctors told his parents he was unlikely to ever talk. Instead, after two years of appropriate speech therapy

Andrew was able to speak at an age-appropriate level and successfully complete first grade. Experiences like Andrew's, along with many other success stories, provide ample proof to speech professionals of the value of their work.

Speech disorders can be very disruptive, but by themselves they are generally not life threatening. This may be one reason why less research is being done on speech pathology than on other, potentially life-threatening diseases. In spite of this, most speech language professionals would agree that people who struggle with speech difficulties can expect at least some improvement in restoring or establishing communication through speech therapy.

Diagnosis

Any speech that interferes with communication, calls attention to itself, or frustrates the speaker and the listener is likely to be a disorder. The diagnosis of the disorder is frequently accomplished through a team effort. Family physicians, neurologists, parents, or teachers who recognize a speech problem typically refer the person to a speech language pathologist, or SLP, who makes the final diagnosis.

The SLP's evaluation includes careful observation, a detailed case history, and a series of special speech and hearing tests. Once all the data has been gathered, the pathologist evaluates and diagnoses the disorder. Part of the diagnosis involves identifying the individual's problem as a speech disorder, language disorder, or both.

The Speech Language Pathologist

SLPs are professionals who are trained to identify and treat communication disorders. They work in a variety of settings including schools, hospitals, rehabilitation centers, nursing care facilities, and private practice.

A career in speech pathology can bring great satisfaction. Eric Sailers, an SLP who works with children in schools, knew he had chosen the right career after helping with a speech therapy research project. "I was so impressed by how [my student's] speech-language skills improved over the course of the research project," he says. "The experience made me realize that I wanted to be an SLP so that I could have a lasting impact on children with communication deficits."[30]

Speech Therapy

Once the diagnosis is made, speech therapy can begin. The speech pathologist now takes on the role of therapist as he or she begins two basic stages of treatment.

During the first stage the speech therapist helps the client identify the problems caused by the disorder. Then, using audio and video recording equipment and mirrors, the therapist shows the client how his or her speech differs from the norm. A client who cannot recognize or is not bothered by his or her disorder is unlikely to put forth the effort necessary to correct it.

Children born with hearing loss need early speech therapy so they will not fall behind in learning.

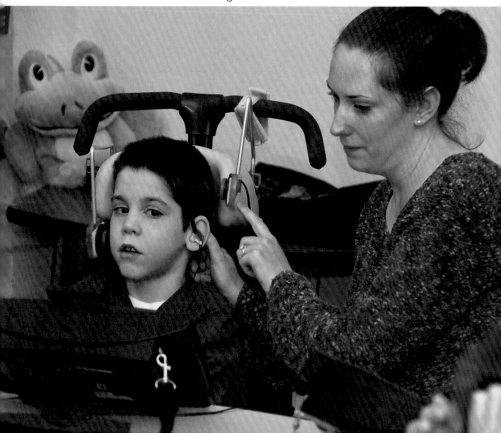

Becoming a Speech Language Pathologist

SLPs generally have a sincere interest in helping others. They work closely with clients to improve speech skills—sometimes developing strong bonds with those they serve. Many SLPs express great satisfaction in being able to help their clients to achieve or restore good speech. To work in this field requires at least a masters degree in communication disorders, a year of supervised work (a clinical fellowship), and a passing score on a national certification examination. In addition, SLPs must meet the requirements for licensure in the states where they practice. Speech pathologists are certified by the American Speech-Language-Hearing Association (ASHA), which represents over 135,000 professionals nationwide. The average SLP annual salary is about $57,000.

Once the client learns to recognize his or her speech errors, the task of correcting them can begin. During this second stage of treatment, the therapist teaches the client new speech skills, using a variety of methods appropriate for the person's s age, case history, and type of speech disorder. The therapist is also careful to enlist the help of those who have close contact with the client, since the success of the treatment depends largely on their cooperation.

Until about age eight, a child is still developing speech habits. When working with children younger than eight, therapy methods are focused on helping them develop appropriate speech while correcting any errors that may be evident. For example, therapists often work with children to pronounce new and more difficult letter combinations while monitoring previously acquired speech skills.

With older patients whose speech is already established, therapists work primarily to eliminate and correct poor speech habits, or in some cases, to help the client learn an entirely new method of speaking. Adult voice disorders require education about the appropriate use of the voice, including information about what *not* to do. However, when adult speech disorders are the result of illness or trauma, therapy is usually aimed at speech recovery. Once the patient is able to demonstrate new skills in a therapy setting, he or she must learn to use them in everyday situations.

Individual Versus Group Therapy

Speech therapy may be given individually or in groups. Generally, patients with less severe speech disorders work well in group settings. Many people feel more comfortable with others who have a similar problem and may improve more rapidly with encouragement from their peers.

Group therapy sessions are usually composed of two or more individuals who are working on the same speech problem. The clients are engaged in many of the same games and speech drills used in individual therapy, but with the added benefit of practicing new speech skills in a safe environment among others who share the same challenges. Group therapy is common in school settings.

Patients with more complex speech problems, such as severe dysarthria or stuttering, however, do best in individual therapy. Individuals who receive personal treatment in one-on-one sessions usually achieve results much faster. During these sessions therapists often direct their clients in tongue exercises and speech drills to help them gain control over the muscles of the mouth, tongue, and throat.

Tongue exercises might include repeatedly touching the tip of the tongue to various locations in the mouth or moving the tip of the tongue across the roof of the mouth from the front of the palate (just behind the teeth) to the very back (where the soft palate is located). Speech drills might include repeated trials of a specific syllable in isolation and then in complete words. Clients are monitored carefully by the SLP, who models the correct pronunciation and provides corrective feedback when necessary.

Speech Therapy Techniques for Children

To the untrained eye a speech therapy session with a child might look more like playtime than work. Therapists often use drill and practice work along with periods of directed play. Sometimes the play is used as a reward for focus during drill and practice, but even playtime is actually therapy. The speech games, flash cards, toys, puppets, "pretend" play, and many other activities are actually therapy techniques specifically tailored to the needs of a speech client. As Darci Truax, an SLP from Gillette, Wyoming, explains, "What the kids don't know is

A speech therapist will often use play during a therapy session.

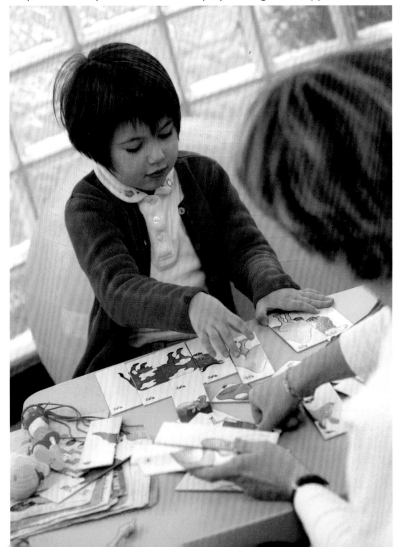

that I am reviewing their mastered words and introducing new sounds and words during their playtime. I have used this technique with children from twenty-four months to twelve years."[31]

Among the other therapy strategies used with children is direct and indirect modeling. Direct modeling is responding to an incorrect sound or word usage by demonstrating its correct use several times. This allows the child to hear the correct word or pronunciation used in normal conversation. Indirect modeling is not prompted by anything the child says but is planned by the SLP to provide repeated practice with a targeted speech behavior. For example, an SLP may bring out a blue box filled with items that begin with the letter b. In this way the child can practice the use of that sound as they discuss first the box and then the items in it.

Sometimes when a child is having trouble with words containing more than one syllable, the SLP breaks the word down into manageable pieces. For example, to teach a child "to say *table*, the therapist may first work with him or her to say *tayo*, then *taybo*, and finally, *table*."[32]

Other speech techniques used with children include expanding and fading. During therapy a child may say something that is not necessarily incorrect but is an incomplete thought with little detail. For example, a child may point to a picture of a well-known nursery rhyme and say, "Cow jump." The therapist may build on what the child says by expanding the original thought to a more elaborated, complete sentence. "Yes, the cow jumped over the moon." Once a child has acquired the necessary speech skills, a therapist may use fading as a way to get the child to demonstrate them: The SLP points to the same picture and says, "The cow . . ." and fades out, allowing the child to complete the thought.

Speech Therapy Techniques for Adults

Speech therapy for adults is usually much more direct and may include focused drills and practice. Many adults go into a therapy situation acutely aware of their own speech deficit and eager to correct it. Some are working to regain speech while

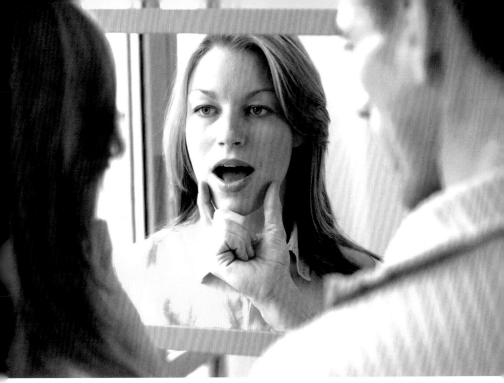

A speech therapist helps an adult client with proper jaw and tongue placement during a therapy session.

others may be tackling a problem left untreated in childhood. In either case, a strong desire to improve communication skills usually prompts adults to work hard to attain their targeted speech behaviors.

Articulation therapy for adults may include many of the same drills and speech activities children do, but without playtime. SLPs focus on helping their clients use proper tongue placement, jaw alignment, and breath control to produce correctly articulated sounds. Repeating sounds over and over, practicing correct mouth movements, and oral exercises designed to strengthen weak speech muscles are all common activities in adult speech therapy sessions.

Certain speech disorders require more specialized approaches. SLPs working with stutterers, for example, may teach their clients to speak in slow motion using short phrases and sentences. They may also work with their clients to avoid words that typically trigger a stuttering episode. These trigger words usually differ from person to person. As the client achieves more fluency the rate of speech is increased. Although electronic devices that provide specially modified auditory feedback are sometimes used to reduce stuttering, most stutterers dismiss them as ineffective.

In the past, patients with Parkinson's disease have not always had the success SLPs would like to see using the traditional speech therapies. Developed by SLPs Lorraine Olson Ramig and Carolyn Mead in 1987 and named for one of the first patients to receive the treatment, the Lee Silverman voice treatment is designed especially for working with Parkinson's patients. The program encourages them to exhale a higher volume of air more forcefully as they speak. The increased effort "pushes" the voice and makes it stronger. Patients learn the new method by attending four sessions a week for four weeks in an intensive regimen that emphasizes forceful speaking. Clinical studies have shown the method to be reasonably successful, although doctors warn it can be harmful to patients with vocal fold damage or disorders.

Therapy for adults suffering from voice disorders differs based on whether the disorder is the result of vocal abuse or damage caused by cancer and its treatment. Voice therapy for adults with vocal nodules teaches the basics of good vocal hygiene and correcting the behaviors that lead to vocal abuse. However, when surgery or cancer treatments have caused differences in the size, shape, and feel of a client's mouth, therapy may also include oral exercises to regain control of weakened muscles or learning to swallow again. Whenever cancer is involved SLPs must often help their clients learn to produce speech in an entirely new way.

Oral Motor Therapy Controversy

Oral motor therapy using nonspeech oral exercises such as drinking through a straw, blowing bubbles, or blowing a horn is a technique often used by SLPs. These exercises are intended to strengthen the muscles for speech production. Those who use it say this therapy aids in speech development. They believe it is especially useful for patients with lisps, CP, dysarthria, cerebral vascular accidents, and cleft palates.

Critics say no scientific studies prove that oral motor therapy works. They point out that the muscles targeted for exercise function differently for speech and nonspeech activities. In spite of the disclaimers many SLPs have traditionally used oral motor therapy in conjunction with other therapy methods.

In 2006 SLP Gregory Lof made a presentation to the American Speech-Language-Hearing Association in which he cited ten different studies that show oral motor exercises have no impact on improving speech. In the wake of this report and other current research many SLPs are coming to the conclusion that oral motor exercises may still have a place in therapy, but not for speech. Many continue to use the exercises for the improvement of eating, swallowing, control of drooling, and other nonspeech activities.

Computer-Based Therapy

Twenty-first-century technology has greatly increased the tools available for speech therapy. Currently dozens of computer-based therapy tools are available to supplement the work of speech therapists. Some are meant to be used independently, others are part of the therapy session and require the presence of an SLP, and still others contain both components.

TinyEYE Technologies Corporation of Canada has developed an online speech therapy application that connects an SLP with a client through any computer with a Web browser, sound card, and camera. This allows speech therapy to take place in remote locations where clients do not have access to an SLP. The therapy methods used are much the same as in a face-to-face therapy session, but SLPs and their clients are connected via the Web. TinyEYE allows parents to be more involved in the therapy process and may increase practice time. TinyEYE already has a commercial stand-alone version which can be customized for individual therapists or institutions, and additional modules are in development.

Another computer-based therapy is a software program called Fast ForWord. Also used as a developmental reading program, Fast ForWord is based on the theory that trouble

Speech Therapy in Schools

According to the American Speech-Language-Hearing Association, over 1 million American students receive speech therapy each year in grades kindergarten through twelve. Most public schools have a full-time speech therapist on staff.

Children who receive speech therapy in school usually attend a class with a group of three or four other students with a similar disorder. The sessions may last from thirty minutes to an hour and occur one to five days a week, depending on the disorder and its severity. A student typically engages in a few minutes of social interaction before starting on an activity tailored to his or her problem area.

As children acquire the skills to overcome their speech disorder, many of them are able to discontinue their therapy and go on to successfully complete their schooling. The satisfaction of achieving this goal creates a sense of pride and confidence that carries over into other areas of the students' lives.

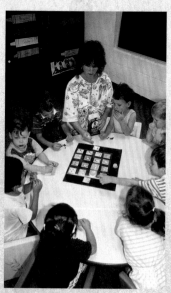

The job market for speech language pathologists is expected to increase well into the twenty-first century. Bilingual therapists will be in demand, especially those who speak Spanish and English. Because speech pathology has the potential to impact so many lives in a positive way, it is a career path certainly worth considering.

In America, over 1 million children receive speech therapy in grades kindergarten through twelve.

processing what they hear is an underlying complication of some people's speech or language disorder. The program uses games designed to slow down and modify individual sounds so that clients are able to distinguish even slight differences. Users are required to accurately duplicate the sounds and provide specific feedback before moving to the next activity. Repeated use increases auditory discrimination. The program requires clients to play the games two hours a day, five days a week. As the client masters the skills at each level, the software automatically moves him or her to the next one. Studies have shown that the program creates language gains of eighteen to twenty-four months in some children. Many researchers, however, believe the results of these studies do not meet scientific standards. They caution that additional testing and study is required to be certain the therapy is effective.

Stroke and cerebral brain injury survivors, victims of degenerative neurological diseases, and children with language-based learning disorders may all be able to benefit from a speech therapy program known as TWIST (Technology with Innovative Speech Therapy). Developed by an SLP in Potomac, Maryland, TWIST features eighteen hours of intensive individualized speech therapy that specifically defines a patient's communication and cognitive strengths and weaknesses. It then matches those strengths and weaknesses with advanced computer software, adaptive hardware, and other helpful devices in addition to traditional therapies. At the end of the program, participants continue their treatment at home using a comprehensive home practice program, software, and other tools targeted to their specific weaknesses. Many participants report extensive progress using the TWIST program, even years after the original onset of their condition.

Music-Based Therapy

Sometimes the best way to rebuild speech capabilities is to look for new pathways in other areas of the brain. Music is one way to do that. When the language center on the left side of the brain is damaged, therapists can tap into the music center on the right side of the brain through a technique called melodic intonation therapy. Although a very low-tech intervention, melodic intonation can produce results in patients as long as nine years after a stroke. The singing and rhythmic tapping that are part of the therapy capitalize on the right brain's unused speech abilities. Former jet pilot Vahan Khoyan, left speechless by a stroke in 2004, was unable to say his own name. After treatment using the melodic intonation technique he is once again able to say, "Hi. My name is Vahan. What's your name?" without missing a beat. Although the signs of his stroke are still evident, his progress with melodic intonation has given Vahan the ability to smile and say, "C'est la vie!"[33] (That's life!)

Another therapy based on the idea of creating new pathways for the production of speech in the brain is a computer-based program called Interactive Metronome. To use the program, clients wear headphones in order to hear a steady beat. Wearing a special glove and standing on a floor mat, the client attempts to produce hand and foot movements in time with specific speech sounds. These activities lead to improved motor planning and sequencing. This helps those with apraxia to order words in a sentence correctly and become more successful with other speech tasks. The exercises are designed to improve the brain's natural ability to repair and remodel itself, a process called neuroplasticity.

Augmentative and Alternative Communication (AAC)

When speech is physically impossible, therapists help their clients learn to use special communication devices. These might include computers with voice synthesizers or other assistive technology. Augmentative and alternative communication, or AAC, includes all forms of communication other than oral speech. Children and adults with severe speech or language problems rely on AAC to supplement their existing speech or replace speech that is not functional. Gestures, body language, sign language, and communication boards are all types of AAC that allow a person with a speech disability to communicate

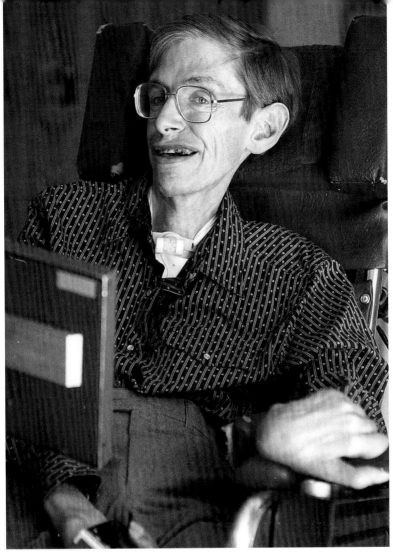

Stephen Hawking, who suffers from amyotrophic lateral sclerosis, uses a hand switch and a computerized voice synthesizer to compose thoughts and translate them into speech.

with people within their sight. Communication boards are special boards covered with symbols of everyday objects and activities. An individual can point to a picture to make his or her wishes known. The Picture Exchange Communication System, or PECS, is an example of using pictures to express desires or thoughts.

A more high-tech means of AAC is an electronic device that produces a voice. Speech-generating devices display letters, words, phrases, or a variety of symbols, allowing the user to construct messages. The messages can be spoken electronically and/or displayed on a screen or a printout.

Stephen Hawking is a renowned scientist, professor, and author who suffers from ALS. He is able to move only two fingers on his right hand and is unable to speak. A computer screen mounted to his wheelchair runs communication software called Voice Text, which produces a robotic sounding voice from text input. Produced by NeoSpeech Inc., this speech synthesizer allows Hawking to press a switch in his hand to compose his thoughts and ideas and have them translated into speech. A hundred years ago Hawking's disease would have rendered him silent within a few years. Thanks to this technology he is able to maintain his "voice" even though he is no longer able to speak.

Except in cases such as Hawking's, AAC devices are intended to supplement speech and can sometimes be phased out as a client's own speech improves. A California mother of a three-year-old boy with expressive language delay found this to be true in her son's case. As she explains, "We started with PECS, then moved to sign language, until finally at twenty-six months he started making some sounds to go with the signs. His therapist was then able to move to more verbal exercises, gradually phasing out signing over the next few months."[34]

Some people reach a point where they no longer feel the need for an AAC device, but others continue to find them helpful in a variety of situations. An autistic man struggling with speech and expressive language disorders is grateful for the assistance his electronic speech device provides. "I like my keyboard," he says. "I've spent my whole life struggling with speech, and I like to have an alternative means of communication. I often feel more comfortable when I use my keyboard because it does not involve the painful and complicated process of speech in addition to language."[35]

While speech therapy is not a miracle cure, most people who deal with communication disorders can be helped by the appropriate therapy. Finding a good SLP is often the first step. Once a diagnosis is made and a course of therapy is determined, hard work and perseverance are the keys to establishing or regaining the ability to communicate freely.

Speech disorders of any kind are a challenge because they interfere with one of the most basic human needs—the need to communicate. Although having a speech disorder is not generally life threatening, it can greatly affect a person's self-image and quality of life. Through speech therapy, many people are able to regain control of their lives by learning new and better communication methods.

Notes

Chapter One: When Communicating Is a Problem

1. Walter H. Manning, "Progress Under the Surface and Over Time," in Nan Bernstein Ratner and E. Charles Healey, eds., *Stuttering Research and Treatment: Bridging the Gap*. Mahwah, NJ: Lawrence Erlbaum Associates, 1999, p. 128.
2. Nancy Lucker-Lazerson, "Apraxia? Dyspraxia? Articulation? Phonology? What Does It All Mean?"www.apraxia-kids.org/site/apps/nl/content3.asp?c=chKMI0PIIsE&b=788447&ct=464133.
3. Quoted in Debbie Feit with Heidi M. Feldman, *The Parent's Guide to Speech and Language Problems*. New York: McGraw Hill, 2007, p. 69.

Chapter Two: Common Speech Disorders

4. Pamela Mertz, "The Way Found Me," International Stuttering Awareness Day Online Conference, 2008 papers. www.mnsu.edu/comdis/isad11/papers/mertz11.html.
5. Walter H. Manning, "Understanding Stuttering as a Gift?" International Stuttering Awareness Day Online Conference, 2008 papers. www.mnsu.edu/comdis/isad11/papers/gift11/manning11.html.
6. Robert E. Owens Jr., Dale Evan Metz, and Adelaide Haas, *Introduction to Communication Disorders: A Lifespan Perspective*, 3rd ed. Boston: Pearson Education, 2007, p. 243.
7. Tina, video post, You Tube. www.youtube.com/watch?v=pqthy-QVT7g.
8. Quoted in Owens, Metz, and Haas, *Introduction to Communication Disorders*, p. 2.
9. Kayla Smith, Kayla's CP Page. http://kaylasmith88.tripod.com/kaylascppage.

10. Megan Hodge, "What Is Neuroplasticity and Why Do Parents and SLPs Need to Know?" www.apraxia-kids.org/site/apps/nlnet/content3.aspx?c=chKMI0PIIsE&b=788461&ct=1990523.

11. Owens, Metz, and Haas, Quoted in *Introduction to Communication Disorders*, p. 367.

Chapter Three: Conditions and Diseases That Cause Speech Disorders

12. Gina Butchin, Cleft Palate Foundation's Story of the Month, May 2009. www.cleftline.org/story_of_the_month/may09.

13. Quoted in The Musical Crematorium, "The Sound of Silence." http://musicalcrematorium.blogspot.com/2004/11/sound-of-silence_20.html.

Chapter Four: Living with a Speech Disorder

14. Quoted in Caroline Bowen, *Speech-Language-Therapy.com.* http://speech-language-therapy.com/lispmail.htm.

15. Loki, video post, You Tube. www.youtube.com/watch?v=DPPIxKKvj1c&feature=related.

16. Manning, "Understanding Stuttering as a Gift?"

17. Ken Steinhardt, "Living with Stuttering," *Orange County Register*, June 25, 2006. www.ocregister.com/articles/living-with-stuttering-1188908.

18. Rose Senerchia, Cleft Palate Foundation's Story of the Month, December 2004. www.cleftline.org/story_of_the_month/dec04.

19. Kendall Tullis, Cleft Palate Foundation's Story of the Month, April 2004. www.cleftline.org/story_of_the_month/apr04.

20. Senerchia, Cleft Palate Foundation's Story of the Month, December 2004.

21. Claire Crawford, Cleft Palate Foundation's Story of the Month, November 2005. www.cleftline.org/story_of_the_month/nov05.

22. Elizabeth J. Bachini, "Share Your Story About Spasmodic Dysphonia," National Spasmodic Dysphonia Association. www.dysphonia.org/support/personal.asp?nav=sup#q2.

23. Quoted in Craig Jarvis, "Triangle Clinics Focus on Voice Disorders," Raleigh (NC) *News and Observer*. www.news observer.com/2766/v-print/story/1022843.html.

24. Quoted in WebWhispers.com, "Laryngectomee Humor." www.webwhispers.org/library/LaryngectomeeHumor.asp.

25. Quoted in WebWhispers.org, "Laryngectomee Humor."

26. Quoted in WebWhispers.org, "Laryngectomee Humor."

27. Quoted in Owens, Metz, and Haas, *Introduction to Communication Disorders*, p. 3.

Chapter Five: Diagnosis and Treatment of Speech Disorders

28. Virginia Pearson, "Speech and Language Therapy: Is It Effective?" *Public Health*, vol. 109, 1995, p. 150. http://download.journals.elsevierhealth.com/pdfs/journals/0033-3506/PIIS0033350605800083.pdf.

29. Pam Enderby and Joyce Emerson, "Speech and Language Therapy: Does It Work?" *British Medical Journal*, vol. 312, June 29, 1996, p. 1658. www.pubmedcentral.nih.gov/pagerender.fcgi?artid=2351353&pageindex=4#page.

30. Eric Sailers, "Interview with Eric Sailers, Speech Language Pathologist," Preschools4All. www.preschools4all.com/speech-pathology-career.html.

31. Quoted in Feit, *The Parent's Guide to Speech and Language Problems*, p. 98.

32. Feit, *The Parent's Guide to Speech and Language Problems*, p. 101.

33. Quoted in ABC7News.com, "Innovative Speech Therapy for Stroke Victims, Speech Learned Through Song," February 23, 2007, http://abclocal.go.com/kgo/story?section=news/health&id=5063560.

34. Quoted in Feit, *The Parent's Guide to Speech and Language Problems*, p. 106.

35. A.M. Baggs, "Autism, Speech, and Assistive Technology," Autistics.org. www.autistics.org/library/spchasst.html.

Glossary

cerebral vascular accident: CVA, stroke, apoplexy; a loss of brain function due to bleeding into the brain.

cognition: Knowledge; includes perception, memory, judgment, and reasoning.

congenital birth defect: A defect or damage that is present at birth.

dementia: Loss of intellectual ability and personality as a result of brain damage.

esophagus: Tube leading from the throat to the stomach.

folate: A compound of the vitamin B complex group found in green plants, fresh fruit, liver, and yeast.

gastric reflux: A backflow of the contents of the stomach into the esophagus.

neurogenic: Caused or affected by the nerves or nervous system.

palate: The roof of the mouth, which separates the oral cavity from the nasal cavity; consists of a bony front portion called the hard palate and a muscular back portion called the soft palate.

postlingually: Occurring after the acquisition of speech and language; usually about age six.

prosthesis: An external or implanted device that substitutes for or supplements a missing or defective part of the body.

resonance: The quality of the sound produced by the vocal chords.

trachea: The tube leading from the larynx to the lungs through which air flows in breathing; also called the windpipe.

vocal breaks: Unintended "cracks" in the voice.

Organizations to Contact

American Speech-Language-Hearing Association (ASHA)

2200 Research Blvd.
Rockville, MD 20852-3289
phone: (800) 638-8255
fax: (301) 296-8580
Web site: www.asha.org

The American Speech-Language-Hearing Association (ASHA) is the professional, scientific, and credentialing association for 135,000 members and affiliates who are audiologists, speech-language pathologists, and speech, language, and hearing scientists.

Cleft Palate Foundation (CPF)

1504 E. Franklin St., Suite 102
Chapel Hill, NC 27514-2820
phone: (919) 933-9044
fax: (919) 933-9604
Web site: www.cleftline.org

The Cleft Palate Foundation (CPF) is a nonprofit organization founded by the American Cleft Palate–Craniofacial Association in 1973 to be the public service arm of the professional association. The mission of CPF is to provide the essential information and research that enhances the quality of life for individuals affected by cleft lip and palate and other facial birth defects.

National Aphasia Association (NAA)

350 Seventh Ave., Suite 902
New York, NY 10001

phone: (800) 922-4622
fax: (212) 267-2812

The NAA is a nonprofit organization that promotes public education, research, rehabilitation and support services to assist people with aphasia and their families.

National Dissemination Center for Children with Disabilities

PO Box 1492
Washington, DC 20013
phone: (800) 695-0285
fax: (202) 884-8441
Web site: www.nichcy.org

The center provides information to the nation on disabilities in children and youth; programs and services for infants, children, and youth with disabilities; IDEA, the nation's special education law; No Child Left Behind, the nation's general education law; and research-based information on effective practices for children with disabilities.

National Institute on Deafness and Other Communication Disorders (NIDCD)

31 Center Dr., MSC 2320
Bethesda, MD 20892-2320
phone: (800) 241-1044
fax: (301) 402-0018
Web site: www.nidcd.nih.gov

One of the National Institutes of Health, NIDCD was established in 1988. Its job is to conduct and support biomedical and behavioral research and research training in the normal and disordered processes of hearing, balance, smell, taste, voice, speech, and language.

National Stuttering Association (NSA)

119 W. Fortieth St., 14th Floor
New York, NY 10018

phone: (800) 937-8888
fax: (212) 944-8244
Web site: www.nsastutter.org

The NSA provides support, friendship, and information to the stuttering community, instilling the sense of self-worth so often missing in the lives of those who battle this disorder. With members nationwide and over eighty self-help support groups in the United States, the NSA provides information about stuttering, increases public awareness of stuttering, serves as a support and advocacy group, and is a referral organization for speech therapy sources throughout the United States.

For Further Reading

Books

Debbie Feit with Heidi M. Feldman, *The Parent's Guide to Speech and Language Problems*. New York: McGraw-Hill, 2007. Written for parents, this is a good guide to speech disorders in children and what the therapy should look like.

Joyce Libal, *Finding My Voice: Youth with Speech Impairment*. Broomall, PA: Mason Crest, 2007. Learn about different types of speech impairments and speech therapy. Along the way meet David, a boy who struggles with stuttering, and Martha, who conquers problems with articulation.

Web Sites

CASLPA Fact Sheets (www.caslpa.ca/english/resources/fact sheets.asp). The Canadian Association of Speech-Language Pathologists and Audiologists have developed a number of excellent fact sheets related to various speech disorders and hearing. The full list of available pdf-formatted fact sheets is available at this address.

Speech Milestones Interactive Checklist (www.nidcd.nih .gov/health/voice/speechandlanguage.asp#mychild). The site provides links to an interactive checklist of speech milestones. Click on the appropriate age bracket to see a list of developmentally appropriate speech skills.

Teens Health: Speech Problems (http://kidshealth.org/ teen/diseases_conditions/sight/speech_disorder.html). This "Speech Problems" article is an overview of speech disorders written for teens. The Web site also deals with a variety of other issues related to teen health.

Young People with Communication Disorders (www .speech-language-therapy.com/adolescents.htm). The site gives an overview of speech disorders in young people written by an Australian SLP for high school and university students and their parents and teachers.

Index

Picture Credits

About the Author

Wendy Lanier is an author, teacher, and speaker who writes and speaks on a variety of topics related to children and parenting. She is married to a college professor and is the mother of two daughters.